TREATMENT PLANNING IN PSYCHOTHERAPY

TAKING THE GUESSWORK OUT OF CLINICAL CARE

SHEILA R. WOODY
JERUSHA DETWEILER-BEDELL
BETHANY A. TEACHMAN
TODD O'HEARN

THE GUILFORD PRESS
New York   London

Library of Congress Cataloging-in-Publication Data

Treatment planning in psychotherapy: taking the guesswork out of clinical care / Sheila R. Woody . . . [et al.].
        p. cm.
Includes bibliographical references (p.   ) and index.
    ISBN 1-57230-805-2 (cloth)   ISBN 1-59385-102-2 (paper)
1. Psychiatry—Differential therapeutics.   I. Woody, Sheila R.
RC480.52 .T74 2003
616.89′ 14—dc21
                                                            2002007022

TREATMENT PLANNING IN PSYCHOTHERAPY

ABOUT THE AUTHORS

Sheila R. Woody is Associate Professor of Psychology at the University of British Columbia and a registered psychologist in British Columbia, Canada. She conducts treatment research on anxiety disorders with colleagues at the Anxiety Disorders Unit at Vancouver Hospital and Health Sciences Center. Dr. Woody was formerly on the faculty at Yale University, where she served as Director of the Yale Psychological Services Clinic and Director of Clinical Training. She has published numerous scholarly papers, including several treatment outcome studies, and a recent book with Peter McLean, *Anxiety Disorders in Adults: An Evidence-Based Approach to Psychological Treatment*. In addition to her research on anxiety disorders, Dr. Woody is committed to promoting and disseminating evidence-based practice of psychological interventions.

Jerusha Detweiler-Bedell is Assistant Professor at Lewis and Clark College in Portland, Oregon. She received her doctorate in clinical psychology from Yale University and completed her undergraduate work at Stanford University. In addition to her work on treatment planning and assessment, she has published on homework adherence in psychotherapy, the relationship between emotional states and physical health, and methods for enhancing health behaviors. Her clinical background includes a term as Assistant Director of the Yale Psychological Services Clinic and a year as a clinical psychology fellow at

McLean Hospital. She is a member of several professional organizations in psychology, regularly presents her work at national conferences, and is the cofounder of the Behavioral Health and Social Psychology Laboratory at Lewis and Clark College.

Bethany A. Teachman is Assistant Professor in the Department of Psychology at the University of Virginia. She received her doctorate in clinical psychology from Yale University and completed her undergraduate work at the University of British Columbia. Her research focuses on change mechanisms in cognitive processing that contribute to psychopathology. Her clinical background includes a term as Assistant Director of the Yale Psychological Services Clinic, and she has worked as a therapist at the Yale Center for Eating and Weight Disorders and at Massachusetts General Hospital. Dr. Teachman is also a contributing author to *Helping Your Child Overcome an Eating Disorder: What You Can Do at Home.*

Todd O'Hearn was previously Director of the Yale Psychological Services Clinic, where he also served on the teaching faculty in Yale's Department of Psychology. His teaching interests include short- and long-term psychotherapy, family systems theory, and integrative approaches to practice. His research interests include the qualitative and quantitative study of community-based interventions. Currently he is developing a private practice in the San Francisco Bay area.

PREFACE

The ideas that gave rise to this book began with a dilemma. In 1999, we were all involved in some way with the graduate training program in clinical psychology at Yale University, as faculty members (SRW), postdoctoral fellows (TO), or doctoral students (JD-B and BAT). The clinical program at Yale strongly emphasizes empiricism. Students learn to conduct high-quality clinical research and to be good consumers of the research literature. Clinical training in the first few years occurs in the context of in-house clinics that rely on empirically supported assessment and treatment strategies.

The dilemma we were facing arose in the later years of training. New Haven offers many terrific practicum opportunities for students who want to gain clinical experience in diverse settings, but the training in many of these clinics involves treatments that have not been tested carefully using controlled research. We wanted to support students in their enthusiasm about the training opportunities, and also to minimize the rift between the empirically based training they received at the university and the clinical practice they would face in the "real world." Essentially, our dilemma was how to help students base their clinical practices on evidence while simultaneously working in settings that did not measure outcomes or rely on empirically tested treatments.

As we began to grapple with this problem, we recognized that our dilemma was not limited to students; conducting evidence-based practice is a challenge for every clinician. The obstacles are clear: high caseloads, poor institutional support for assessment, inaccessibility of the clinical research literature, and relative homogeneity of theoretical orientation in tested treatments. This book represents our attempt to create a system to address these challenges: planning and assessment in clinical care (PACC). This system outlines a treatment planning method guided by reliable information about each client, providing a step-by-step organizational structure for identifying and prioritizing client problems, conceptualizing phases of treatment, establishing concrete treatment aims, and measuring progress toward those aims. At the same time, PACC is flexible enough to be applicable to a wide variety of clinical populations and to be useful for practitioners in all disciplines of mental health care. PACC makes no assumption about the type of treatment being offered; it will work with any treatment approach for which measurable goals can be established.

After we wrote an initial draft of our ideas for the PACC system, we began to apply its principles in practice. We also recruited colleagues to test the approach and provide us with feedback. Since that time, we have used the PACC method for several years ourselves, even as the members of our group scattered to various parts of North America. Overall, the PACC approach has been used by clinicians with a variety of experience (ranging from first-year graduate students to professionals with 10 years of experience), in a variety of settings (including graduate training programs, private practice, and inpatient and partial hospital programs), with clients presenting a wide variety of problems.

Evidence-based practice is the foundation of the PACC approach. We strongly believe in the utility of the scientific method for determining which treatments work and for whom. Accordingly, we provide as many resources as possible to assist clinicians in keeping up to date on the research literature, recognizing the time limits imposed by full-time practice. However, we also believe that evidence-based practice does not rely only on randomized controlled trials. The main purpose of this book is to provide clinicians with an organized system of science-based tools for formally evaluating the degree to which therapeutic goals are being met. Because only a portion of clients resemble participants in clinical trials, a fully relevant model of evidence-based practice must use evidence obtained locally from each client.

Many clinical practice books are organized so that clinicians can select a single chapter that addresses a pertinent clinical problem. This approach is sensible in many ways, because each chapter is relevant to a given subset of clients. Our book is not like that; it is designed to be valuable for nearly every client, regardless of presenting problem or even the theoretical orientation of the therapist, so that it is less useful to read isolated chapters. Read the whole book. The first chapter sets out the rationale for the PACC approach. Chapters 2 through 6 are like a series of building blocks, each describing one element of the approach in detail. Many case descriptions are sprinkled through these chapters as we illustrate the challenges and benefits of applying each component. Finally, Chapter 7 follows a single case through several phases of treatment, illustrating how all the pieces fit together in a system that provides high-quality information to guide treatment planning, and also discusses some of the ethical implications and potential applications of the PACC system beyond private practice.

Of course, we have many people to thank for their assistance in completing this project. We greatly appreciate the contributions of Susan Mirch-Kretschmann and John Perez in the early stages of developing this project, as well as the administrative assistance of Lucy McCullough at its conclusion. Thanks also to the many people at McLean Hospital and Yale University who shared ideas with us and tested the PACC method in their own clinical practice, especially Ana Cragnolino, Shauna Dowden, Jim Grossman, Philip Levendusky, Edmunde Neuhaus, Matt Nock, Nilly Mor, Eshkol Rafaeli, and Monica Thompson. Special thanks are due to Alan Kazdin for his encouragement and advice. We thank James Shetler from Yale University's Social Science Libraries and Information Services for his assistance in compiling the list of websites and databases that appears in Chapter 4, as well as the Saint Mary's College Library online resources for their list of book references. Finally, we thank Lori Charvat, Brian Detweiler-Bedell, Brian Nosek, and Holly Garcia O'Hearn, our respective spouses and life partners. Without their support, tolerance, and willingness to sacrifice time with us, this book would have remained simply a good idea.

SHEILA R. WOODY
JERUSHA DETWEILER-BEDELL
BETHANY A. TEACHMAN
TODD O'HEARN

CONTENTS

TREATMENT PLANNING IN PSYCHOTHERAPY

CHAPTER 1

THE PACC APPROACH TO TREATMENT PLANNING

Successful treatments rarely occur by chance. Rather, they follow from a series of thoughtful decisions in which clinicians predict how they can best help clients achieve treatment goals. Clinical decision making is an exciting and challenging process that requires therapists to integrate science and creativity to meet the unique needs of their clients.

Take the case of Kelly, a 32-year-old married woman with no children, who was diagnosed with generalized anxiety disorder (GAD). She sought treatment for "problems with worry and anxiety," exacerbated by her husband's recent change in jobs and her own lack of satisfaction in the day care center where she had worked for 6 years. Kelly's therapist initially tried to teach her anxiety reduction and worry control strategies but found that she was not particularly responsive to these interventions. Specifically, Kelly did not practice the suggested techniques between sessions, and she came into each session with a new "crisis" that required immediate attention. Kelly's crises ranged from financial to interpersonal to existential matters. The therapist kept note of the "urgent issues" that Kelly raised each week. Over the course of a month, Kelly had discussed her fears of being in debt, inability to have children, drinking alcohol, having sex, experiencing grief, dying in an accident, being deserted by her husband, getting sick, caring for her mother, and developing a neurological disorder. Two months into treatment, Kelly had not experienced any relief from her worries or her anxiety. The therapist began to feel frustrated with the scope and unpredictability of Kelly's concerns and was similarly frustrated by Kelly's noncompliance, yet was unsure about whether to continue in the same vein of treatment or to switch to a new approach.

This book is about applying an evidence-based approach in the everyday world of clinical practice. We describe and illustrate a structured set of tools to address the pressures and challenges of treatment planning. We call this set of tools the PACC approach: Planning and Assessment in Clinical Care. Our aim is to provide a straightforward system for setting and monitoring the progress of treatment goals, independent of specific therapeutic procedures. The world of psychotherapy has changed dramatically in the last 10 years, with pressures from many directions to amend the way therapists practice. The motives behind these influences are laudable, such as improving the quality of psychosocial interventions, but many of the proposed elements of an evidence-based approach have proven unfeasible for routine clinical practice.

To help clinicians practice in today's mental health care arena, we have developed a structured approach that uses the best science available, yet remains flexible and spontaneous, and operates relatively independently of theoretical orientation. The PACC method of treatment planning is both cost-effective and relevant for practice, regardless of the specific therapy approach. In this chapter, we begin by discussing some of the professional issues that motivated us to develop the PACC system. Our primary focus was to bridge the gap between research and practice with an evidence-based approach that is practical for clinical work.

In recent years, more and more mental health professionals identify their theoretical orientation as eclectic (Lazarus, Beutler, & Norcross, 1992; Patterson, 1989), reflecting their desire to integrate multiple treatment approaches. However, most clinical trials use relatively pure (and intensive) forms of a single treatment, and therefore offer little help to the practicing clinician who wishes to fashion a treatment plan composed of several different approaches, such as behavioral activation and couple therapy. As a result, some skeptical observers have argued that eclecticism results in therapists who know a little about a lot of different approaches, leading to casual treatment planning that is poorly justified by research or theory. Hans Eysenck (1970) characterized eclectic treatment as "a hugger-mugger of procedures, a galli-maufry of therapies" (p. 145) that lack empirical support and a defensible rationale.

In contrast, we believe that the word "eclectic" does not have to connote a haphazard approach to treatment planning and delivery. Although no widely accepted definition of eclectic psychotherapy has emerged, we like the early definition proposed by English and English (1958), who described eclecticism as "the selection and orderly combination of compatible features from diverse sources, sometimes from incompatible theories and systems; the effort to find valid elements in all doctrines or theories and to combine them into a harmonious whole" (p. 168). A clinician who embraces this definition may eschew rigid allegiance to a single theoretical orientation, be that psychodynamic, neurobiological, cognitive-behavioral, family systems, or any other method.

There will never be enough resources to conduct clinical trials comparing all possible permutations of treatment plans for all types of clients who seek help. Even the large and expensive studies, although important in establishing treatments that are effective in general, fail to provide sufficient guidance to the individual clinician formulating a treatment plan for a specific client with multiple problems. We saw this situation as a challenge to develop tools that enable flexible, eclectic treatment planning that simultaneously draws from outcome research and responds to the unique needs of individual clients.

The shift to a more eclectic approach can be credited partly to the development of specific techniques that are effective for treating specific disorders, such as panic and phobias (Garfield, 1996). Even as early as 1976, some psychologists began using the term "prescriptive psychotherapies" to describe an approach that attempted to match clients with treatments likely to work (see Goldstein & Stein, 1976); more recently, researchers and clinicians have revived support for this prescriptive approach (Beutler & Harwood, 1995). The real challenge for clinicians who value an evidence-based approach remains how to plan treatment for individual clients, knowing that these well-studied treatments do not work for every client, and that many client problems have not been subjected to careful study.

The main emphasis of PACC is repeated assessment to guide treatment planning while engaging the client (as appropriate) in collaborative goal setting and progress evaluation. We present an overview of the PACC approach in the rest of this chapter and demonstrate how this model addresses many of the concerns about manualized treatments. The remaining chapters in the book provide details on each component of the PACC system.

PACC: GOING BEYOND RANDOMIZED CLINICAL TRIALS

Although psychotherapy researchers have been working to develop a base of evidence for the effectiveness of various treatments, our field has not truly integrated research and treatment, as envisioned in the scientist–practitioner model. Applying science in practice is not easy, even for those who believe that first-line approaches should be empirically supported treatments, when they are available. Finding out which treatments have good research support for the client's problem is only the first step. After that, the therapist must figure out the specifics of the treatments and how to conduct them. PACC depends partly on treatment studies and draws heavily from basic research methods in a system that attempts to maximize a clinician's objectivity and flexibility in treatment planning.

Results of randomized clinical trials are undeniably an important foundation for general treatment planning. Although it is true that these studies do not closely resemble typical clinical practice, they do show the potential of a given intervention—how the intervention performs under very favorable conditions (e.g., clear focal problem, highly supervised and specifically trained therapists). Furthermore, these clinical studies endeavor to demonstrate conclusively that a given treatment, rather than some other variable, is responsible for observed improvements. Because of the degree of confidence that these studies permit, treatments demonstrated to be efficacious in randomized controlled trials should automatically be considered candidates for treatment approaches when they are available (see Chapter 3).

However, evidence-based practice cannot rest entirely on these clinical trials. Treatment planning clearly needs something beyond theoretical orientation (which no longer fully guides practice) and outcome literature (which guides researchers but has limited utility for practice). Pressures for accountability and the recognized value of scientifically supported practice indicate that evidence (data) should drive decision making in clinical practice. This imperative pertains not only to the selection of treatments but also to the whole treatment course, which includes documentation of progress for individual clients. Not long ago, single-case experimental designs were advocated for use with every client, but this approach proved too burdensome (Kirk, 1999). Notwithstanding, data that evaluate each client's progress can form the basis of successful, accountable practice. PACC enables clinicians to do this efficiently and without necessarily deviating from their theoretical orientations.

For the most part, practitioners judge whether clients are improving and goals are being met by asking questions or gleaning information from material the client spontaneously presents during the session. In the general course of practice, assessment occurs only at the beginning of treatment (usually with unstructured interviews). Clinicians, like most people, feel fairly confident in their judgments; unfortunately, confidence is not related to accuracy of judgment. On the one hand, research has demonstrated that clinicians are overconfident in some of their judgments, such as which clients will remain in therapy and what behaviors are expected from a normal subject (Garb, 1994). On the other hand, clinicians are underconfident when classifying clients using formal assessment procedures; that is, clinicians classified clients more accurately than they suspected when using formal assessment methods (Garb, 1994).

Establishing treatment objectives for each client and then assessing progress toward these objectives is the key to a feasible system of evidence-based practice. Individualized and continuous assessment brings the scientific approach down to the level of the individual and guides treatment planning. PACC aims to extend the concept of eclectic practice, proving particularly useful when the research shows conflicting results about which treatment is most helpful or when the pattern of problems a particular client brings to therapy has not been specifically researched. Clinicians are left to their own creativity (drawing from their general theoretical understanding of psychopathology, human development, and sociology) to come up with specialized treatment plans in these cases. Regular measurement using reliable and valid instruments provides the eclectic clinician with the means to decide when to maintain an ongoing intervention and when to switch to a new approach.

Evidence-based practice, therefore, rests on knowledge of the scientific findings (to guide the selection of a treatment approach, when possible) and sound measurement of client progress (to determine if the selection is a good one for the particular client). Another important element is a willingness to throw out an earlier hypothesis or conceptualization should it prove faulty. After a client's problems are evaluated and the therapist has become educated about (or refamiliarized with) interventions that have been tested for a given problem and client demographics, he or she is in a position to formulate an accountable treatment plan.

PACC: ENHANCING ACCOUNTABILITY

"Accountability" refers to answering questions about the value and integrity of one's work. When used to refer to nonprofit organizations, "accountability" generally means offering publicly available evidence that charitable donations are used responsibly and in the ways that donors would reasonably expect. Business types often speak of accountability to stockholders, indicating the responsibility of a business to demonstrate that it is upholding a fiduciary duty to maximize return on investments. In both cases, accountability refers to good faith efforts to ensure that money is well spent and that expectations for its use are fulfilled.

Although these are positive and reasonable aspirations from the perspective of the investor, the term "accountable" can also have negative connotations. Many mental health providers cringe when they hear the word "accountability." To them, it implies an assumption that without being monitored, they would be unaccountable—essentially selling snake oil. Let us focus instead on the positive aspect of accountability, that of documenting value. We believe psychotherapy is a worthwhile endeavor that can make an enormous difference in the lives of our clients. The challenge is to articulate what we expect those differences to be and to measure whether our expectations are met.

The PACC system can facilitate this process by providing a structure for specifying aims and measuring progress toward them. Note that accountability always references the time and resources required to meet the goals in light of reasonable expected outcomes; no one expects a Hunger Relief Agency to end a war, remove corrupt politicians, and produce rain, in addition to feeding starved people. Similarly, it is unreasonable to expect therapists to "cure" their clients' bodily symptoms of anxiety, help them get a promotion, and secure for them an ideal romantic relationship, in addition to reducing the frequency of panic attacks. Clearly specifying goals that are appropriate for the client's situation can help make it easier to document accountability, because reasonable goals are explicit, encouraging all interested parties to use the same yardstick. Furthermore, providing a plan and data to support treatment decisions may minimize the likelihood of lawsuits following disappointing outcomes or conflict among interested parties (Morrison, 1984).

GUIDING PRINCIPLES OF OUR APPROACH

Sackett, Richardson, Rosenberg, and Haynes (1997) describe evidence-based practice as the conscientious, explicit, and judicious use of current best evidence in making decisions about the care of individuals. Hallmarks of evidence-based practice include use of an individualized assessment in combination with well-researched treatments to formulate (and reformulate) a treatment plan. One of the components of expert clinical judgment is the ability to recognize the limitations of subjective judgment and to make the best use of available empirical evidence (Wilson, 1998). As we have argued, this evidence includes not only published research on treatment outcomes for a given *group* but also data gathered through careful assessment of *individual* clients.

In developing a feasible, theory-neutral model of evidence-based practice for routine practice, we have relied on seven guiding principles reflecting our philosophy that ideal clinical care should draw on a combination of theory, research, and evaluation.

1. Different approaches to psychosocial treatment are likely to have merit and be effective, even those that have not been thoroughly tested. Drawing from several theoretical approaches for treatment planning is valued, so long as treatment planning is guided by regular evaluations of the impact of treatment.
2. Each client is an individual who requires treatment based on a thorough assessment consisting of clinical interviews and approaches with documented reliability and validity. In the absence of such approaches, assessment is grounded in theory and undertaken with the goal of formulating and modifying a treatment plan.
3. Assessment is ongoing throughout treatment and is used to evaluate (a) whether treatment is helping the client accomplish his or her goals, and (b) whether any characteristics of treatment should be changed. The client, a partner in this process, is informed of the results of the evaluations.
4. The means and goals of treatment are explicit, written, and agreed upon by client and therapist.
5. When choosing treatment strategies, clinicians should look

first to treatments that have been empirically tested for the problems their client presents. When no outcome research is available to guide the selection of a treatment approach, or when clinicians feel that their particular client is not well represented (economically, culturally, etc.) among the research samples, the selected strategy should be grounded in theory where possible, and the impact of this strategy should be evaluated regularly.

6. Clinicians should continually evaluate the impact of treatment even for those treatments that have been well established in psychotherapy research. Identifying lack of change is just as important to treatment planning as observing that change has occurred.

7. Treatment planning is best accomplished with an iterative, flexible approach. When evaluation indicates that treatment is not promoting progress toward the goals of therapy, the approach is changed or referral to another setting is considered.

OVERVIEW OF THE MODEL

As we mentioned earlier, PACC is a model that focuses on assessment as an ongoing endeavor to shape treatment planning throughout the course of therapy. Although we have discussed psychotherapy research as a basis for treatment planning, our focus is more on steps the individual clinician can take to maximize accountability (to oneself and others) and monitor treatment progress for individual clients. The steps of the PACC model are described in detail in the following chapters, but here we provide a brief overview.

The PACC model consists of three main components: a *Problem List*, a *Treatment Plan*, and a *Progress Review*. The Problem List is formally developed during the initial evaluation, but new problems are added as they become apparent during any stage of contact with the client. The Treatment Plan has three elements: *aims*, *measures*, and *strategies*. Treatment planning is divided into phases, each representing a focus on a specific subset of client goals, which we refer to as aims. At the beginning of each phase of treatment, the therapist identifies what aims will be the focus of the phase, chooses measures by which progress toward the aims can be evaluated, and plans specific intervention strategies designed to promote attainment of the aims. Improvement on these aims is evaluated at the end of each treatment phase through a Progress Review. The number of phases of treatment will vary depending on the client's set of presenting problems and the degree of improvement across these problems.

A central objective of the PACC model is to offer procedures to promote accountability that are feasible to implement in routine practice. The intended beneficiaries of accountability are not managed care review panels (although many of the suggested procedures do correspond to paperwork required by third-party payers). Rather, we have endeavored to develop a system by which the clinician can approach treatment planning in an individualized yet structured way. The PACC approach allows the clinician to feel confident about whether the treatment is working, and it encourages the client to be a partner in evaluating the progress of therapy. Furthermore, the PACC system of treatment planning is orientation-neutral and *independent of any particular treatment approach*. The theoretical assumptions rely on the value of specifying aims, measuring progress toward those aims, and planning interventions. In the PACC approach, treatment goals can reflect the full range of aims targeted in clinical practice, including broad goals (e.g., improve marital communication) and specific aims (e.g., expand listening skills). The Treatment Plan is reviewed on a regular basis and changed as often as necessary to promote successful outcomes on specific aims.

WHAT ARE THE BENEFITS OF THE PACC APPROACH?

Although the scientist–practitioner approach has been promoted in psychology training programs for 50 years, there have been few feasible models for mental health providers to actually implement scientifically sound practices. We designed the PACC approach to address practitioner concerns and to respond to the contemporary pressures in the world of practice. Some of the main practitioner concerns reviewed by Addis, Wade, and Hatgis (1999) include the therapeutic relationship, the complexity of client needs, competence and job satisfaction, treatment credibility, and feasibility.

Therapeutic Alliance

Therapeutic alliance is of central concern to many treatment approaches, and all practitioners rely on the relationship as a vehicle for conducting psychotherapy. The PACC system is relevant for the working alliance in two primary ways: first, PACC is entirely compatible with a partnership approach to treatment in which the therapist and client collaborate to identify problem areas, establish goals, and acknowledge progress; second, the therapeutic relationship itself may be one of the problems the therapist chooses to enumerate on the Problem List. For example, a client's resistance to the idea of treatment is a relevant problem even though the client may not endorse it as such. If the therapist does not address the resistance and join with the client, he or she is unlikely to accomplish other therapy aims. In this way, the therapeutic relationship can be a relevant aim (often in the earlier phases of treatment). Thus, the PACC approach is designed both to foster a positive alliance and to make the therapy relationship an explicit focus of treatment if it has gone awry.

Individualized Client Needs

Targeting client needs on an individualized basis is one of the primary strengths of the PACC model. Although clients with similar diagnoses obviously share some basic problems by definition, the details vary quite a bit from one client to the next. The iterative nature of the PACC model is sensitive to the clinician's evolving understanding of the client's unique set of problems. Although manualized treatments may address some of the items on a client's Problem List, these formalized approaches are designed for the modal client with a particular diagnosis. Most clients have extra issues that need attention, as well as new problem areas that emerge over time, once the therapeutic relationship has developed.

For example, one of our clients came to treatment because of his fear of flying. He had been afraid of flying for several years, but his fear had become an issue in his life only recently, when changes in his work situation resulted in increased travel. Being accustomed to using treatment manuals, the therapist's first thought was to use a tested manual for the treatment of simple phobia. When the client arrived for his initial evaluation, however, the therapist discovered that he was also afraid of crossing bridges, driving, and going through tunnels. The element that seemed to unite all of these problems was this client's increased sensitivity to physical signs of anxiety. His response to sensations of anxiety was to cut short the anxiety-provoking activity and to avoid it in the future.

The therapist changed her mind about the specific phobia treatment manual, feeling that its focus was too narrow, and she began to think instead of applying a protocol for treatment of panic disorder. Although many elements of this approach would be helpful, the trouble was that this client denied ever having experienced a panic attack, rendering many parts of the manual (and the suggested measurements of progress) irrelevant. Therefore, although a cognitive-behavioral approach seemed like a good first strategy, the therapist was not able to rely on any single manual in its entirety to design her treatment plan.

Instead, the therapist improvised the Treatment Plan from elements of several tested approaches and used the PACC system to check repeatedly whether her strategy was impacting on the client's avoidance and anxiety. She used previously established questionnaires to evaluate the client's difficulty tolerating sensations of anxiety (e.g., Anxiety Sensitivity Index; Peterson & Reiss, 1987) and his avoidance of a range of situations (e.g., Mobility Inventory; Chambless, Caputo, Jasin, Gracely, & Williams, 1985). However, she also formally asked the client for ratings of his level of fear of particular bridges and tunnels in the area, as well as his fear of taking flights to various destinations that were relevant to his life (i.e., fear hierarchy). In this way, she used measurement of the client's presenting problems to determine whether her individualized Treatment Plan was showing success.

Therapist Competence and Job Satisfaction

Clients who have multiple problems, particularly those who have life situations or personality styles that raise new problems every week, are particularly challenging to the therapist's sense of competence and job satisfaction. Maintaining a therapeutic focus with such clients is a challenge that most treatment manuals simply ignore, and prioritizing and balancing the various problems are not issues that treatment research has so far examined. Clearly, the PACC model cannot make it easy to treat multiproblem clients, but we do believe the approach offers several tools to help manage the difficulties.

Kelly (introduced at the beginning of this chapter) is an example of a client who appeared to benefit from the application of the PACC approach. About 8 weeks into Kelly's treatment, the therapist (overwhelmed by all of Kelly's "crises") began to implement the PACC approach to reformulate her case and to attempt a fresh perspective. Accordingly, the therapist consolidated a list of Kelly's concerns and presented this list to Kelly in session. In looking at her Problem List, Kelly commented that her therapist "really was paying attention to what I've been talking about." The therapist, in turn, used the Problem

List to identify a pattern in Kelly's problems. Specifically, almost all of Kelly's "crises" involved issues that made her feel that she was out of control. Using this theme, the therapist first talked more clearly with Kelly about how treatment might help her, based on the revised case conceptualization. For example, the therapist suggested strategies such as having Kelly assess the extent to which she could control events, accept that life is somewhat unpredictable, and recognize that she had the ability to tolerate some lack of control.

The therapist then found appropriate strategies for reaching the treatment aims and measured Kelly's progress on these aims more systematically. In addition, the therapist took advantage of the collaborative nature of the PACC approach by enlisting Kelly's help in the therapeutic planning process. The therapist found that Kelly was far more likely to stay on task in session if she had played a role in choosing the agenda for the session. In addition, any time that Kelly brought a new concern into the session, the therapist simply added it to the Problem List and asked Kelly to assess whether this new problem could be fit into the aims of the current session, or if it should be set aside for another point in treatment. Kelly's therapist found this approach highly rewarding, mainly because it enhanced the collaborative nature of the therapeutic relationship, helped to maintain treatment focus, increased Kelly's motivation, and led to a more systematic evaluation of whether the treatment was helping Kelly with her problems.

As illustrated in this case example, we have found in our own practice with the PACC system that actually writing out the Treatment Plan helps to keep the focus clearly in mind. As will become clear in later chapters, we consult the Problem List when developing the plan for each phase of treatment. Before we began to use the PACC system formally in practice, we had mentally developed a problem list for each client, as do most therapists. However, we discovered that taking the time to write things down provides clarity of purpose that amply rewards the time we invest. We found that committing the Treatment Plan to paper helps us to clarify our formulation of how the client's various problems fit together and organizes the strategies to address them, thereby helping to structure case conceptualization.

Clients can also benefit from the collaborative process of enumerating and prioritizing their problems. As was true for Kelly, this process can help clients to maintain focus and increase their motivation. When a client raises a new problem, the therapist can immediately add it to the Problem List and briefly assist the client in deciding whether to continue with the plan as previously agreed or shift focus to the new problem. In this way, many new problems can simply be added to the list as elaborations. Thus, even without shifting the treatment focus, the client has the opportunity to register the problem as important enough to add to the list. This approach of considering a new problem and deciding to address it later (in deference to more pressing current problems) is compatible with some other treatment approaches, such as problem-solving therapy (D'Zurilla, 1986).

Finally, the most direct contribution of the PACC method to therapists' sense of competence and job satisfaction may come from the increased confidence that they are providing effective treatment that follows from monitoring clients' improvement. As we describe in later chapters, graphing client progress on measures administered repeatedly is not time consuming when one has mastered some basic computer skills. We feel a strong sense of satisfaction in seeing the client's improvement displayed on a graph; charting progress is definitely worth the time it requires. Most clients also respond very well to seeing these graphs.

Credibility of the Treatment Plan and Client Satisfaction

Credibility reflects the client's and the therapist's faith in the treatment rationale and the plan for addressing the client's problems. At first, clinicians are likely to feel self-conscious when trying out a new approach. Although clinicians will undoubtedly feel awkward when first implementing procedures associated with PACC, we have found the evidence-based approach quickly improves treatment credibility and client satisfaction. Most practitioners find that they are already implicitly incorporating many of the elements of the PACC approach in their standard practice, so they only need to add a few elements and make the steps more explicit.

Client satisfaction can be assessed at two levels (Shaffer, 1997). The typical way to evaluate client satisfaction involves asking clients about their global sense of the treatment and its value. Organizations that are interested in this type of measure typically ask clients to complete a questionnaire near the end of therapy. The PACC method leads to a deeper sense of client satisfaction by helping clients to develop a clear sense of their aims in treatment and evaluate whether those goals are being met. Most clients come to therapy knowing something about their problem(s) but with little idea how to conceptualize their goals for treatment. Because a primary focus of the PACC approach is clarifying aims of treatment and measuring progress toward those aims, there is enormous potential for clients to see eye to eye with the therapist about treatment goals and intervention strategies.

Feasibility

Practitioners are usually pressed for time, so evidence-based practices need to be efficient and cost-effective. The PACC method takes much longer to read about than to do! When we began to implement PACC procedures in our clinical work, we dreaded sitting down to write the Treatment Plan, because it seemed like an enormous task. Once we actually made ourselves do it, we were surprised to find that about 15 minutes was required per treatment phase (not per session) for each client. As we became more skilled, that time was reduced further. In-session time is also quite small, ranging from none (for those therapists whose approach is less collaborative and whose clients complete questionnaire measures in the waiting room) to whatever time the therapist chooses to allot for a Progress Review. Having spent the time to organize the treatment plan, we also found that we subsequently spent less time preparing for each session, because we had a written road map to guide agenda setting within each treatment phase.

The PACC system is also easy to learn. Because it is applicable to a variety of therapy orientations, therapists can rely on their present skills while moving toward an evidence-based approach. Supervised experience is not required to develop competence in the PACC method, although consulting with one's colleagues about measurement ideas may be helpful to those practitioners who have little experience in monitoring progress.

The PACC system is also recommended for clinicians working in environments that are already committed to an evidence-based approach. Even when therapists use a well-tested treatment manual or follow highly structured treatment guidelines, specifying goals and measuring progress toward those goals is beneficial. No psychosocial intervention is so powerful that it resolves every client's problems, and it is useful to keep track of which problems are improving and which remain unchanged. Furthermore, measurement facilitates good treatment planning even for clients with prototypical problems for which well-established treatment manuals are available.

A few years ago, one of us was treating a client with panic disorder and mild agoraphobia. The treatment setting encouraged the use of manualized therapies, so the therapist selected the revised therapist guide from *Mastery of Your Anxiety and Panic* (Craske, Meadows, &

Barlow, 1994). This straightforward manual outlines a 15-session treatment plan. After only a few sessions, however, the client experienced a sudden improvement. Having heard the therapist's explanation of the physiological basis of sensations of anxiety and engaging in a behavioral experiment with hyperventilation, the client no longer feared that his anxiety would rise indefinitely until he lost his mind. Although most clients require more experience with these concepts before they feel willing to trust them, this particular man quickly improved. He no longer saw a need to avoid situations, such as church or restaurants, because he felt confident that anxiety sensations were uncomfortable but not dangerous. Had the therapist forged ahead with the treatment manual without measuring progress, she may not have known that the client was ready for tapering and termination much faster than she had anticipated.

Documentation and Informed Consent

Explicitly identifying client problems, articulating a Treatment Plan based on specific aims, measuring progress toward those aims, and responsively modifying the Treatment Plan based on the data are all practices that enhance ethical and legal standards of practice. The explicitness of the approach toward treatment planning facilitates fully informed consent, particularly if clients themselves are involved in gathering information relevant to their treatment goals. Furthermore, the paper trail generated by the model is an excellent record-keeping tool for systematically documenting treatment decisions, which in turn provides legal protection to clinicians.

In working with clients who are litigious, involved in the legal system, or who have a history of antisocial (e.g., violent, threatening) behavior, it is particularly important to have substantive documentation supporting the clinical decision-making process. For example, Elton was a 50-year-old father of four whose wife had recently requested a separation and filed for a restraining order because of Elton's increasingly intense episodes of rage. In the 3 weeks prior to seeking treatment, Elton had totaled three cars, punched his fist through the wall of his bedroom, broken numerous pieces of furniture, and threatened his wife and children with a baseball bat. Elton sought treatment for his uncontrollable anger, hoping to "win back" his wife and family.

Elton's treatment team had not reached a consensus as to his psychiatric diagnosis; he was being treated pharmacologically for bipolar disorder but had rule-out diagnoses of both borderline and antisocial personality disorder, as well as a possible neurological abnormality. Working with Elton was challenging for the therapist, in part because of his propensity to fabricate elements of his own life history and the details of his current struggles. However, Elton was motivated to restore the trust of his wife and children and his symptoms of rage appeared to be ego-dystonic. When presented with the choices involved in treatment planning, Elton required considerable guidance, but he was ultimately an active participant in the process. He helped the therapist to identify problem domains, and he was able to admit to problems reported by his wife and by his coworkers that he had not endorsed during the initial intake.

Elton and his psychiatrist were able to use the PACC approach as a structured way to document his problems and form a treatment plan. Specifically, Elton agreed to work with his clinician to develop an impulse control plan. In working on this short-term goal, Elton learned to identify the triggers of his rage, coping strategies, alternative behaviors, and interpersonal supports. Moreover, Elton agreed to check in with his psychiatrist (by leaving phone messages), reporting the number of times he felt an impulse, the content and triggers of the impulse, and his response(s). In working with clients like Elton, clinicians may worry about their own liability in the event that their client were to act out an impulse (especially an impulse to hurt himself or another person). In using the PACC approach, practitioners have substantial documentation testifying to the extent to which the client has been targeting problem areas, learning new skills, and practicing these skills.

WHAT THE PACC APPROACH IS NOT

The PACC approach has features related to manualized treatments, program evaluation, practice guidelines, and treatment research, but it is distinct from each of these approaches. Furthermore, the PACC approach is not time consuming or expensive, characteristics that would greatly limit its use in routine practice.

Manualized Treatment

Although our book may be conceptualized as a manual for treatment planning and assessment, the PACC approach is not a manualized treatment. Manualized treatments provide specific guidelines for treating particular problems, and treatment manuals are often quite detailed, providing session-by-session outlines of what to do. Research on manualized treatments is grounded in the assumption that clinicians can simply take treatment manuals off the shelf and apply them to their own work with clients. The expectation is that treatment manuals or protocols ensure that the tested intervention is consistent across therapists. Nonetheless, the use of treatment manuals does not eliminate individual differences in therapist success (Luborsky, McLellan, Woody, O'Brien, & Auerbach, 1985).

Debate has raged across psychology (e.g., Havik & VandenBos, 1996), social work (e.g., Gambrill, 1999), and psychiatry (e.g., Glazer, 1994) with regard to the advantages and disadvantages of applying treatment manuals in practice. By and large, clinicians have resisted this model of evidence-based practice. We believe one major reason for this resistance has been the way evidence-based practice has been formulated and presented. Manuals, although representing a decided advance in specifying treatments and promoting training in new approaches, do not sufficiently reflect the complexity of treatment. As Wilson (1998) wrote, "Empirically-supported, manual-based treatments are good, but not good enough" (p. 367). Although these treatments are preferred based on their scientific support, clinical innovation is still required.

Many clinicians are convinced that they already offer effective treatment and so feel little motivation to go to great lengths to learn new interventions. Furthermore, reflecting their own doubts, some practitioners worry that clients will not find a new approach credible or acceptable. Because of these potential shortcomings, many therapists are concerned about the feasibility of an evidence-based approach that relies on manualized treatments. Treatment manuals are unlikely to specify the order, combination, or amount of intervention for individual clients with complex problems. Furthermore, in many clinical settings, practitioners are required to provide extremely short-term treatment (to keep costs down), making rigid, session-by-session protocols unrealistic. In addition, the administration in mental health disciplines rarely supports high-quality continuing education. As a result, there is often little financial assistance for mental health professionals who seek formal opportunities to build new skills.

The debates on evidence-based approaches to mental health practice have often focused on manualized approaches to treatment, about which practitioners have many legitimate concerns. But evidence-based practice entails more than manualized treatments. We see manualized treatments as a cornerstone of an evidence-based approach such as PACC, but a cornerstone does not a building make.

Program Evaluation

Program evaluation is similar to the PACC approach in that both evaluate whether goals are being met, without taking pains to establish the basis for inferring that the intervention caused the observed change (Chen, 1993). The central function of program evaluation is simply to provide a valid assessment of the effectiveness of a program. Among the mental health disciplines, social work and community psychology are most commonly involved in program evaluation. Approaches to program evaluation range from methods that resemble tightly controlled randomized trials to those that emphasize external validity, with the aim of facilitating pluralistic decision making.

The PACC approach can potentially be modified to facilitate certain types of program evaluation, but evaluating the effectiveness of an entire program is not the purpose of the PACC system. The central functions of the PACC model are to structure treatment goals and provide a valid assessment of the degree to which treatment goals are being met. The unit of analysis is the individual case (meaning an individual client, family, or couple) and the individual provider(s) responsible for treatment, rather than the entire program.

Program evaluation is an important endeavor, but two main weaknesses limit its utility for treatment planning: First, clinicians in many settings simply have no access to program evaluation services because they have historically been available mostly for government-funded programs to evaluate whether a program is achieving the goals for which it is being funded; a second weakness of program evaluation as a guide for treatment planning is that it provides feedback *after* treatment is finished. Program evaluation addresses whether the intervention program is meeting overall goals for the community it serves. Treatment planning for individual cases more optimally involves an iterative process of setting goals, providing an intervention, measuring progress toward the goals, and reevaluating both the goals and the intervention strategy in light of the ongoing measurement. Program evaluation is too general and occurs too late in the process to be useful for this purpose.

Practice Guidelines

Practice guidelines essentially offer a scientifically derived template for treatment planning with clients who have specified problems (Kirk, 1999). The main difference between the PACC approach and practice guidelines is flexibility. By necessity, practice guidelines are confined to commonly occurring problems that typically fall into major DSM diagnostic categories. In general, these guidelines do not address the specific aspects of a problem that are most troublesome for a particular client, or additional problems that may be related to the diagnosis but are not diagnostic symptoms (e.g., marital strain for a depressed client). Furthermore, practice guidelines often fail to offer recommendations for treatment planning in the event that the best researched strategies are ineffective for a given client. The approach we describe encourages clinicians to use innovative strategies in circumstances such as these and allows them to be confident that they are monitoring the case as carefully as possible.

Treatment Research

The goals of treatment research are to test whether a given treatment is capable of effecting change in clinically relevant problems or to describe the processes by which those changes are effected. Accordingly, the design of treatment research includes many controls to rule out alternative explanations for the observed effects. Whereas these controls permit stronger inferences, they limit the generalizability of treatment research to clinical work in the field. PACC does include some of the features of treatment research, mainly involving the use of reliable and valid measurement, but it is less restrictive. The clinician's goal typically is not to pinpoint the source of client change but to encourage the process of change by whatever means necessary. Hence, we do not discuss issues of internal validity as a feature of PACC. Instead, we focus on specifying what needs to be changed, how to know if it has changed, and what to do if it has not. Whether the putative effective ingredients of the intervention are responsible for affecting the change is another question. Here, we are simply interested in the degree to which change is occurring.

TIME AND COST

Individual clinicians can implement the PACC system even in an environment that is indifferent to evidence-based practice because the approach does not require organizational support. While coordinating efforts across clinicians can confer some additional benefits, no committee is required to use these principles for treatment planning. Likewise, monitoring outcomes in a systematic way can involve costly service improvements, but the PACC model is simple and inexpensive, requiring no fancy database system. Furthermore, we have purposely designed PACC to overlap considerably with the paperwork that is already required in many accredited settings, such as community mental health centers or Veterans Administration (VA) hospitals.

Using instruments that are in the public domain (i.e., free to photocopy), we estimate that the direct cost per client to implement the PACC system is about $0.25 per session. The cost increases when one uses instruments that must be purchased, but there are many instances when free measures are available. In our own experience using PACC across various settings, we find that (after becoming familiar with the approach) we spend an average of 5 minutes of in-session time and 5 minutes of therapist time for each session. This time is not distributed evenly across sessions. In some sessions, no time is spent on treatment planning or measurement. In others, the time will be limited to asking clients to take a questionnaire home and complete it before the next session. In preparation for other sessions, the therapist may spend 15 minutes planning aims, measures, and strategies. However, this preparation typically guides treatment for several sessions, resulting in a good investment of time.

CHAPTER 2

DEVELOPING
A PROBLEM LIST

The Problem List is a tool for managing and prioritizing the client's difficulties. As such, it is not a one-time list developed at the beginning of treatment and never revisited. We consult and update our Problem Lists repeatedly throughout treatment: when new problems arise, when progress is observed on treatment aims, or when new information prompts a shift in the case conceptualization. Not all of the problems on the list will be addressed by treatment goals; some problems may relate to the client's environment or personality style, without being direct targets of treatment.

Procedures similar to the creation of the Problem List are required as a part of treatment planning in many settings such as VA hospitals and many publicly funded community mental health centers. In these settings, the Problem List can be incorporated into the required documentation with little effort. The main task involved in making the Problem List a useful tool for treatment planning is to survey comprehensively the potential domains of concern for the client, then to prioritize and effectively narrow the list to guide a given treatment phase. In this chapter, we discuss the domains of functioning that should be included in the Problem List and also consider the role of case formulation and various factors related to prioritizing the problems on the list. Some of our comments in this chapter may be more relevant to new clinicians than to seasoned practitioners.

WHY FORMALIZE THE PROBLEM LIST?

The process of developing the Problem List is not a new one for most clinicians. Assessment is always the first step in seeing a new client, and clinicians usually develop a list of the client's problems, even if the list is simply a mental one. The case notes usually include mention of at least the presenting problem(s), although often in fairly global terms. If developing an implicit list of the client's problems is already standard practice, then what is to be gained by taking the time to refer to a checklist, write an explicit Problem List, and review all or parts of it with the client? Making an explicit list can positively affect the client, the therapist, and the client–therapist relationship. Because careful practitioners already cover many of these activities, the additional time investment is minimal.

If the Problem List is developed collaboratively, there are often clear benefits for the client, because the list can concretize and organize problems that previously seemed vague and overwhelming. Specifying the client's problems in clear and relatively operational terms can make them seem more accessible and potentially more amenable to change, which is particularly important for clients approaching their first experience with psychotherapy. Also, parsing large, diffuse problems into subsets of more specific problems fosters hope and sparks motivation.

Neophyte therapists may notice that developing a Problem List helps them to feel less overwhelmed and can help them to structure session time efficiently, particularly in the initial stages of therapy. Rather than simply asking clients to talk about their problems, the clinician can guide the discussion to specific areas and focus on the most relevant information. By relying on a checklist to make sure the bases are covered, therapists can begin to distinguish important from nonessential information for treatment planning.

Even experienced clinicians may find value in writing an explicit Problem List. While using a checklist may seem like a strategy that would be valuable only for clinicians who are new to therapy, a checklist can reduce the probability of missing important problem domains. In a multidisciplinary treatment team setting, the Problem List can incorporate areas assessed and monitored by professionals in nursing, psychiatry, psychology, and social work. Using the Problem List in this way can help the numerous caregivers organize their efforts and highlights the contributions made by professionals across disciplines. We have included a blank Problem List form in Figure 2.1.

	Client endorsed?
1.	
2.	
3.	
4.	
5.	
6.	
7.	
8.	
9.	
10.	
11.	
12.	
13.	
14.	
15.	
16.	
17.	
18.	
19.	
20.	

FIGURE 2.1. The Problem List.

Experienced clinicians will certainly want to supplement our checklist with domains that are important in their particular area of practice. Using such an enriched checklist can avoid the problem of getting into a mental rut before treatment even begins. When a client is referred with a particular diagnosis, for example, clinicians often develop expectations about what types of problems will usually be associated with that diagnosis. These expectations can be helpful guides, but they sometimes lead therapists to shortcut the assessment process. (Note that this problem may also occur when the client has a particular ethnic background, reports certain historical experiences, or has any other feature that may invoke stereotyped thinking.) Garb (1994) has pointed to examples of clinical decision making that are influenced by the biases that characterize general human thinking patterns. Using a checklist can help the clinician to gather information that has the potential to support *or refute* initial hypotheses about the client.

As treatment proceeds, the Problem List suggests a clear agenda for the course of treatment, encouraging structure and organization across sessions. This element is particularly critical for therapists working under the constraints of a limited number of sessions in which to help the client. On the surface, it might seem that looking at a whole Problem List would be overwhelming when only a few sessions are available. Nothing can assuage the discouraging feeling of having a client who needs 20 sessions but whose coverage permits only four. However, the Problem List can at least help to highlight priorities and facilitate solution-focused creative thinking.

We have also found that the Problem List aids in case formulation, which we discuss in some detail later in the chapter. Outlining all of the pertinent issues at the outset helps the therapist to develop a coherent story about the client and her problems, integrating what at first appear to be disparate pieces of information. This kind of holistic understanding can lead directly from the Problem List to a plan for treatment and ongoing assessment of the problem areas. In addition, noting how the problems appear to be interrelated can help the therapist anticipate barriers to treatment. For example, a depressed client might benefit from engaging in positive activities, but if he also has serious financial problems, then he will not do well with strategies that cost money. In this case, the therapist would want to focus on going for a hike as an enjoyable activity, rather than going to the theater or to a professional sports event.

Finally, creation of the Problem List can enhance the quality of the client–therapist relationship from the outset. Gathering an exhaustive list of problems offers the chance for the practitioner to empathize with the client right away. Furthermore, by assuring clients that treatment strategies and constructive solutions can be generated for each problem, the practitioner can convey a sense of confidence and hope, thereby helping clients to build their own positive beliefs about therapy. We have experienced the creation of the Problem List as an opportunity to set a precedent for collaborative discovery early in treatment, thus laying the foundation for a good working alliance. Some therapists also find it helpful to create the Problem List with a view toward formalizing a therapeutic contract.

DOMAINS OF FUNCTIONING:
A BIOPSYCHOSOCIAL PERSPECTIVE

The specific items covered on the Problem List will undoubtedly vary depending on the clinician's viewpoint and style. Nevertheless, most clinicians want to take into account the client's acute difficulties as well as the broader context of his or her life. Creation of the Problem List begins by focusing on indicators that are most relevant to the client's presenting problem(s). For example, some of the client's symptoms of depression, such as suicidal ideation and uncontrollable crying, may be more bothersome or disruptive to functioning than other symptoms, such as irregular eating. The clinician is also encouraged to consider broader difficulties that may be associated with the client's core problems. Here, the therapist may take into account positive behaviors that the client does not do often enough (e.g., specific social skills or engaging in pleasant events), as well as maladaptive behaviors or distorted thinking patterns. In addition to considering elements related to the client's presenting problem(s), the Problem List should be augmented with more general concerns following a thorough biopsychosocial assessment. This broad assessment can often clarify the degree to which the presenting problem affects multiple domains of the client's functioning, or the ways in which secondary problems may influence treatment for the primary concerns. We consider these domains within two basic rubrics: (1) problems associated with the presenting complaint, and (2) problems that may have a bearing on treatment planning, without necessarily being a focus of treatment.

The Presenting Complaint and Related Problems

Treatment outcome studies traditionally judge therapy success primarily in terms of reduction in distressing symptoms, often those linked to a specific diagnosis. More recently, the concept of outcome has been broadened to better reflect the type of clinical assessment that occurs in practice, which includes evaluation of not only the client's symptoms but also his or her interpersonal and role functioning (Lambert, Okiishi, Finch, & Johnson, 1998). Certainly, the Problem List will cover distressing or maladaptive symptoms, including motoric, physiological, emotional, and cognitive or ideational problems (Paul, 1974).

In addition to the various aspects of the presenting problem, the Problem List should include related problems associated with the physical environment and the client's social life (Paul, 1974), especially those factors that appear to elicit or facilitate the maladaptive behavior (Goldfried & Davison, 1994). For example, obsessive–compulsive hoarding behavior can lead to reduced living space and angry reactions from family members. Contextual factors are also included if they appear to set the time or place for the occurrence of the problem behavior. For example, marital disputes may serve as a trigger for abuse of alcohol, or feelings of abandonment may serve as a trigger for self-injurious behavior such as cutting. Finally, it is important to consider environmental factors that either reduce the occurrence of the problem behavior or promote the behavior. For example, a child may not have temper tantrums in the presence of an older brother who models alternative coping methods, and an agoraphobic client may be willing to go certain places while in the company of a trusted friend. Other, related factors might be cognitive in nature (e.g., expectations); even physiological factors (e.g., pregnancy) may influence the expression of the problem behavior.

Enumerating aspects of the presenting problem in specific and concrete terms provides the first opportunity for the clinician to operationalize the client's problems. The next steps, which are described in Chapters 3 and 4, involve establishing therapeutic aims and measuring progress toward those aims. Conceptualizing the client's problems in somewhat measurable terms for the Problem List facilitates those subsequent steps in treatment planning. Although one could simply list a diagnostic label as one of the entries on the Problem List, each client experiences symptoms (e.g., of depression) in unique ways within a particular context. Taking an individualized approach to the Problem List involves specifying the bothersome or disruptive aspects of depression for each particular client. For example, Francine, a 32-year-old divorced mother of two, was referred by her family practitioner because she had been depressed for several years and was not responding to antidepressant medications. Her Problem List began with attention to the two aspects of her depression that were the most troubling (see Figure 2.2).

Francine initially described her problem as "I've been depressed my whole life." The therapist helped her to enumerate the specific problems that fell into her description of "depression." Figure 2.2 shows Francine's Problem List, which was developed in stages as her

	Client endorsed?
1. Suicidal ideation	√
2. Feelings of sadness	√
3. Frequent absences from work	√
4. Loneliness	√
5. Generalized anxiety	√
6. Fatigue	√
7. Insomnia	√
8. Weight gain	√
9. Feeling worthless	√
10. Ambivalence in role as mother	
11. No role models for consistent and warm parenting	√
12. Unstable work history	
13. Court involvement related to custody dispute	√
14. Frequent arguments by telephone with ex-husband	√
15. Not confident of daughters' love	√
16. Inconsistent visitation with daughters	√
17. Few social contacts	
18. No exercise	√
19. Poor diet (mostly fast food)	
20. Alcohol and tranquilizer abuse	

FIGURE 2.2. Problem List for Francine.

therapist completed the initial evaluation. Items 1–9 were generated in relation to Francine's complaints about her depression. Although she endorsed all of the problems (1–9), she did not generate them all without prompting from the therapist. For example, Francine certainly lamented the reduced income that resulted from her frequent absences from work, but she did not initially frame this as a problem. Rather, she saw her absences from work as further proof of what a "worthless basket case" she was.

Other Relevant Problems

In addition to the client's presenting problems and cultural considerations, clinicians often evaluate factors that may be problematic in relation to the selection and implementation of intervention strategies. For example, a clinician may wish to include the client's spouse in certain parts of the therapy, but if the client has kept the problem secret from the spouse, this will be an impediment. As another example, being able to point to specific, concrete examples of when the problem behavior occurs facilitates cognitive-behavioral interventions, but if the client cannot do this, then raising awareness will need to be taught as a first step (Goldfried & Davison, 1994). A client who says, "I was depressed all night after I heard what used to be 'our song' on the radio," provides a concrete example of a depression trigger, but some clients can only say, "Last night I was really down."

Other factors to consider are clients' standards for their own performance; clients with overly high expectations may become discouraged with slow but steady progress. As Goldfried and Davison (1994) point out, the availability (or lack) of appropriate role models or social partners is also an important consideration in treatment planning. The client's own social characteristics are also important. These characteristics represent relatively stable traits that may interact with treatment as assets or liabilities; they may also interact with the problem behaviors (Paul, 1974). Characteristics such as ambivalence to change or poor motivation also can be included on the Problem List.

The client may also face problems related to interpersonal functioning, as is often the case for those with social anxiety or anger management problems. Similarly, risky behaviors are often the direct focus of treatment for individuals with impulse control problems; in other circumstances, they may be monitored without intervention (e.g., if the client is not ready to change). Finally, some clients never raise issues of spirituality and moral development, whereas others approach psychotherapy with problems in these domains as their primary focus.

To continue with the earlier example the therapist saw that Francine had some ambivalence about her role as a mother. Francine described her own mother as emotionally distant and self-absorbed when interacting with her, but warm and engaged with the grandchildren. Thus, although the relationship between Francine and her mother was cordial, the therapist viewed Francine's mother as a poor role model for helping Francine develop a more consistent parenting style toward her own children. When the therapist gently inquired about Francine's view of her mother as a role model for consistency and warmth, Francine agreed with the therapist's observation and noted that she had never really thought about this before. These items are noted in Francine's Problem List as items 10 and 11 in Figure 2.2.

Minimizing Cultural and Other Biases

Another important consideration for the creation of the Problem List is the cultural background of the client, beyond just ethnicity. Hays (1995) advocates thinking more broadly about diversity in assessment to become conscious of client age or generational differences, physical challenges, religion, ethnicity, social status, sexual orientation, and indigenous heritage, as well as nationality and gender. Even when thinking about ethnicity alone, the impact on clinical practice is substantial. Ethnic minorities make up approximately 25% of the American population, but only 5.1% of psychologists are ethnic minorities (Hammond & Yung, 1993). At present, we have a limited understanding of how cultural background may alter the course of treatment. Nevertheless, the variance in cultural norms and beliefs about what constitutes health versus dysfunction emphasizes the importance of practitioners considering the influence of culture (broadly speaking) when creating the Problem List.

In trying to understand the biases embedded in popular assessment approaches, it is important to recognize the assumptions that guide our practice. We all work from a particular framework, influenced in part by our cultural background, upbringing, and personal experiences. Because we are typically guided by the dominant culture's beliefs about what constitutes "normal," the major classes of cultural bias that typically emerge are biases in diagnosis (in the direction of stereotypes associated with a given population) and unreasonable judgments of a problem's severity (Lopez, 1989). To guard against these biases, Lopez (1997) encourages clinicians to be wary of either over- or underpathologizing.

On the other hand, it is critical to be aware of the potential impact of the client's background and unique environment. Some cultural issues may pose problems for the client, such as acculturation differences between generations in an immigrant family. Other cultural issues may be more subtle or diffuse, such as clients struggling with their sense of ethnic identity. Due to lack of knowledge about a particular culture, therapists may be unwittingly biased about what constitutes a problem. Sex role stereotyping is one case in which this could happen; loyalty to family culture and wishes is another.

For example, Michelle, a first-generation Asian American college senior working toward a double major degree in human biology and psychology, sought treatment for mixed anxiety and depression, triggered in part by her confusion over career choices. Michelle's dream was to become a social worker, but her parents expected her to go to medical school. Her therapist's initial reaction was to put items such as "difficulty with assertiveness" and "overreliance on parental approval" on the Problem List. However, after listening carefully to Michelle's description of her cultural upbringing, her relationship with her parents, and the importance of her heritage, the therapist reconsidered these "problems" and decided instead to focus more directly on Michelle's problems with anxiety management and social isolation.

One does not want to stereotype by assuming that cultural or other norms apply to a particular client without first checking the client's degree of acculturation or sense of cultural/minority identity. One useful measure of acculturation is the Stephenson Multigroup Acculturation Scale (SMAS; Stephenson, 2000). Stephenson defines "acculturation" as the extent to which the client is immersed in the "dominant" (in this case, United States) society compared to his or her original or "ethnic" society. The SMAS assesses the client's cultural immersion in domains ranging from language and food to media and social interaction. The scale has good reliability and validity, and can be especially helpful at the outset of treatment, when the therapist is trying to determine the impact of unique cultural variables on a client's functioning, and to determine the appropriateness of selecting culture-specific assessment or intervention approaches.

Another useful measure of acculturation is the Vancouver Index of Acculturation, which based on the assumption that acculturation is bidimensional, with separate elements corresponding to heritage and mainstream culture identification (Ryder, Alden, & Paulhus, 2000). More information and a copy of the scale can be obtained at *www. psych.ubc.ca/~dpaulus/del/research/viapage.htm*.

In addition to assessing the client's degree of acculturation, it may also be helpful to consider culture-specific service delivery issues. Dana (1993), who created an instructive list, which we have modified and included in Table 2.1, describes this list as a reminder "to be alert to each one of these possible issues prior to developing a plan for assessment that includes not only choices of tests/instruments but the desirability of client-shared decisions for test administration and subsequent use of findings" (p. 207). Dana encourages therapists to revise and update this list of service delivery issues in order to best match the concerns or considerations relevant to their particular client population.

TABLE 2.1. Cultural Identity Considerations

Group identity/cultural orientation (check one):

____	Traditional	Culture _____
____	Nontraditional	Original culture _____
____	Bicultural	Original culture(s) _____
____	Multicultural	Original culture(s) _____

Possible service delivery issues (check all that apply):

____ Language preference differs from that of clinician (client's first
      language: _____)

____ Ability of assessor to communicate assessment findings (language
      competence or style)

____ Desire for assessment results

____ Ability to understand results (possible conflict with beliefs)

____ Mental health services are unacceptable

____ Somatization is preferred symptom expression

____ Self-concept includes "others" with priority

____ Family may make ultimate decisions

____ Acceptability of the service provider

____ Culture-specific presenting problem

____ Adequacy of DSM for assessee

____ Other _____

Note. From Richard H. Dana, *Multicultural Perspectives for Professional Psychology.* Copyright 1993 by Allyn & Bacon. Adapted by permission.

The first item on Dana's (1993) list, and one of the most important initial considerations in treating culturally diverse clients, involves the degree to which the clinician is comfortable with the client's primary language. One of our clients, Mia, a 26-year-old woman from Estonia, moved to the United States at age 15. She attended a public high school and then went to a community college. Prior to her psychiatric difficulties, she had been working full-time as a manager of a local coffee house. Over a period of 3 months, Mia's increasing withdrawal and isolation led her to miss work and break off contact with friends. Finally, Mia was picked up by the local police, who found her wandering along the side of the interstate highway a mile from her home. Mia was hospitalized, and members of her treatment team believed she was experiencing a psychotic episode characterized by both visual and auditory hallucinations.

It was difficult to assess her functioning, in part because her English was extremely poor. There were no clinicians on the staff who spoke Estonian, which made it challenging to determine the extent of her problems. The treatment team finally was able to contact Mia's mother, who lived on the opposite coast of the United States. Mia's mother agreed to travel to the hospital to assist her daughter, and she worked together with the treatment team to assess Mia's language abilities. As it turned out, Mia's native Estonian was just as fragmented and unintelligible as her English. Mia was treated with antipsychotic medication and over the ensuing months made a significant, although not total, recovery.

Mia's case highlights some of the challenges of treating a client with a different ethnic and cultural background. Sue (1998) developed three guiding principles to promote "cultural competency." First, he notes the importance of being "scientific minded," which reflects the essence of the PACC approach, in that he advocates the development and testing of culture-relevant hypotheses by gathering data. In this way, therapists are less vulnerable to the risks of ignoring the role of culture or stereotyping a specific person. Second, by developing skills in "dynamic sizing," the practitioner can judge when to generalize and inclusively reflect group norms (i.e., when to think about the client as a member of a larger social group with unique cultural standards) versus when to individualize (i.e., when to focus on the client as an individual who makes choices distinct from those expected given his or her cultural background).

Livingston (1999) provided an excellent example of a case in which group norms and the behavior of the individual were important considerations. He described a 14-year-old girl whose parents immigrated from Cuba with their own parents in the 1950s. The daughter was brought into treatment for being inattentive, "daydreamy," and easily distracted. The client's mother described her as "verbally impulsive in the extreme," unable to keep any thoughts to herself:

> Her teachers complained principally about her uncompleted work, but her parents' chief complaint was her "disrespect," as evidenced by her impulsive statements. These were especially shocking and humiliating to them now, since her mother's parents were living with the family and always commented that they "never would have allowed your mother to talk to us that way." The child acknowledged feeling guilty when she said something hurtful but said she did not know how to control this behavior.... Her parents explained that something had to be done, because they were unwilling to tolerate her disrespect, which was simply "not acceptable in our culture." A brief course of individual therapy emphasized techniques for situational control of verbal impulses and avoidance of conflicts or even contact when she was especially irritable. Family therapy, including the grandparents in some sessions, emphasized information about ADHD [attention-deficit/hyperactivity disorder], impulsiveness and rebound, and it reframed disrespect as requiring a level of intent which is not necessarily present in an impulsive utterance. After a few sessions, their family life was considerably more peaceful. (pp. 1592–1593)

As Livingston (1999) pointed out, perceived disrespect is a concern that is not limited to any single ethnic group. Extended families can exacerbate problems of cultural dissonance among immigrant families, because the older generations may be more "traditional." Many older members of the family have come to expect to be treated in a particular way, consistent with norms from their native culture, and generational changes may not be welcome. Livingston also described this case as illustrating that interested parties (e.g., children, teachers, parents) may differ considerably in what they think the targets of treatment should be. He suggests that obtaining chief complaints from all involved parties may be particularly important if there is reason to suspect discordance between cultures at home, school, or work; among peers; and in the community.

A third consideration to keep in mind, according to Sue (1998), is that by being prepared (e.g., reading what is known about assessment of a particular group), one can become proficient in dealing with the cultural group. Before administering assessments to a client, we recommend doing a quick search of the literature to determine if a more appropriate tool is available (either in the primary language of the client or with norms for the client's group). Resources for finding these tools are included in Chapter 4, and clinicians interested in learning more about multicultural psychotherapy can turn to several recent sources (Hays, 1995; Miller, 1999; Organista & Muñoz, 1996; Rogler, Malgady, Costantino, & Blumenthal, 1987; Sue, 1998; Sue & Zane, 1987).

AN OUTLINE FOR BIOPSYCHOSOCIAL ASSESSMENT

Table 2.2 includes an outline that may be a useful reminder of different biopsychosocial assessment domains that should be considered when creating the Problem List. The list is fairly exhaustive, but it focuses on general problems that would be evaluated for clients with a wide variety of presenting problems. Naturally, each presenting problem area will have its own more specific items that should also be included. As examples, the Behavioral Health domain usually includes weight for clients with eating disorders; Sexual Functioning would be added for clients with sexual problems or for distressed couples. Readiness to change and other motivational factors are likewise not included on this list, simply because its purpose is to focus on domains of functioning.

Our outline can be used several different ways. Experienced clinicians who already have an efficient initial assessment procedure may wish to use the outline as a double check to ensure that their current system covers all the appropriate bases. Other clinicians may already be familiar with analogous models, such as Lazarus's BASIC-ID (1997), which also helps to structure client assessment. Alternatively, the biopsychosocial assessment outline provided here could be used as a checklist assessment areas beyond the focal symptoms or the presenting problem. Using this method, one might prepare a copy of the list as a reference to provide some structure for initial interviews.

Problems involving potential *injurious behavior* (i.e., physical harm to self or others) are particularly important to evaluate for inclusion on the Problem List. Suicidal ideation or self-mutilation may or may not represent an immediate crisis or relate directly to the present problem. However, these issues are always problematic behaviors and should be included on the Problem List even when they are present in mild forms.

In addition to features of the presenting problem and harm-

TABLE 2.2. Domains for Consideration for the Problem List

Domain	Specific issues to assess
Injurious Behavior	Suicidal ideation or behavior Homicidal ideation or behavior Self-mutilation
School/ occupational functioning	Attendance Performance Disciplinary action Overall job or school stability Financial status related to occupational functioning
Family functioning	Relationships with all family members (e.g., parental, marital) Family crisis/trauma Parenting skills (e.g., disciplinary issues with children)
Other interpersonal functioning	Adjustment to interpersonal life stressors (e.g., issues of loss, separation, letting go) Quality of social supports Frequency of social contact Excesses and deficiencies in social skills
Behavioral health	Physical fitness and exercise Nutrition and eating habits Medical history (including medications) Appropriateness of health-seeking behavior Use of legal drugs (e.g., caffeine, nicotine, diet medications)
Risky behaviors	Alcohol abuse Illicit drug use Unsafe or inappropriate sexual behavior Gambling Thrill seeking
Culture, spirituality, and moral development	Cultural influences and difficulties Involvement with religious institutions Existential questions and challenges Moral dilemmas and issues

related issues, daily functioning is also important. *School or occupational functioning* should be assessed, including attendance, performance, disciplinary action, overall job stability, and corresponding financial status. Continuing with the example of Francine, we noted earlier that missing work was a problem listed on her Problem List. Francine worked as a home care nursing aide and in recent months had missed at least a shift a week at her job. She had also been fired from several jobs in the past few years because of poor attendance.

Family functioning was also problematic for Francine. Her relationship with her parents was satisfactory, but she was involved in a custody dispute with her ex-husband over their daughters (ages 9 and 11). Francine lived alone (her husband had custody of the children) and saw her daughters every other weekend. However, she often asked her parents to care for them on the weekends, when it was her turn to have the girls. Francine was afraid that her ex-husband would turn her daughters against her, and she felt powerless to "make them" love her. She and her ex-husband argued frequently by telephone.

Although of less concern to Francine, her *other interpersonal functioning* also appeared to be poor. She reported having few friends and no romantic relationships. Because the therapist felt that the absence of social contacts was a problem to be monitored even though Francine did not endorse this as a serious concern, it was noted on her Problem List (item 17) but not checked off as "client endorsed."

In the area of *behavioral health*, Francine was also having difficulty functioning. In the last several years, she had gained a lot of weight and led a very sedentary lifestyle. Her diet consisted primarily of fast food, and she reported feeling continually stressed out. Medical conditions would be important to note in the domain of behavioral health, but in this case, Francine denied any current problems. Although she did not use the word "abuse" herself, Francine abused alcohol frequently and minor tranquilizers occasionally. In assessing *risky behaviors*, the therapist noted that Francine reported driving and going to work under the influence of alcohol.

Items 10 through 18 were added to Francine's Problem List after her therapist assessed problems of functioning in addition to the symptoms previously included on the list. Notice that the therapist did not indicate Francine's endorsement on several items. Francine viewed her unstable work history as a misfortune but did not see it as relevant to her depression, or as a problem to address in psychotherapy. Likewise, she did not see anything wrong with her diet or use of alcohol and tranquilizers.

Francine's Problem List is very long (it ultimately contained 20 items), but this is not unusual for complex clients who present with multiple diagnoses or difficulties in role functioning. The idea of creating such a comprehensive list is not to overwhelm the client or the therapist, but to help clarify the multiple interacting issues that cause distress in the client's life. This list can then be used to prioritize the aims for treatment, so the therapist can be confident that a critical problem domain is not being overlooked. There is no expectation that every problem will be addressed in therapy, and certainly not in a single phase of treatment.

Language of a Good Problem List

We have discussed the content of the Problem List, including content related to the presenting problem and to personality or contextual issues that the therapist believes will impact on treatment. In addition to comprehensively covering the client's problems, a good Problem List will be arranged in such a way that it facilitates subsequent steps in the PACC model, including case formulation, intervention planning, and measurement of progress on the problem. Based on their different backgrounds and training, the therapist and the client will often use different language to describe each problem. The challenge in a collaborative approach is to strike a good compromise, so that the client's meaning is preserved while the problem is described in terms that will be useful for treatment planning. For example, one of Francine's first complaints about her current situation was "I'm lazy." With more questioning, the therapist discovered that Francine was referring to her frequent absences from work, as well as her general fatigue. Construing "lazy" as problems with attendance at work, motivation, and sleep captured Francine's problems in a way that facilitated the therapist's case conceptualization, as well as the measurement of the problems.

It is also be important when creating a Problem List to distinguish problems from goals. Sometimes when clients are asked to describe their problems, they instead describe their dreams for a better future: "My problem is that I want to move out of my parents' house, have a steady job, and show everyone that I am doing something productive with my life." It may be tempting to turn the client's goals immediately into problems: (1) living in parents' home, (2) unemployment, and (3) lack of productivity. In many cases, however, some of the meaning in the client's stated goals is lost in this direct translation.

In such a situation, we encourage therapists to ask the question, "What is preventing my client from achieving his goals?" In the previous example, a better understanding of the client's goals may actually imply a somewhat different set of problems: (1) lack of social supports outside of the family, (2) difficulty maintaining a normal sleep–wake schedule, and (3) beliefs that he is incompetent and a failure. Careful assessment of the meaning of the client's stated goals and use of the case formulation may help in creating more useful language for the Problem List.

Collaboration in Forming the Problem List

Developing and maintaining the Problem List is a flexible process in terms of the degree to which therapists involve clients, ranging from fully collaborative to solely managed by the clinician. How much to involve the client in the creation of the Problem List depends on therapist style as well as client characteristics. For some therapists, one of the first tasks of treatment is to collaborate with the client in generating a list of all the problems she or he would like to address in therapy. The therapist and client may then prioritize the problems together, deciding which to tackle first. For therapists working in a very collaborative style, any reconsideration of the Problem List will involve a discussion with the client, and the client and therapist are likely to look over the list together.

Consider this example of a social worker using a very collaborative approach with a client, Lucia, an administrative assistant in her 30s. Lucia had recently completed a phase of treatment in which she had successfully worked on accepting the end of a long-term abusive relationship. During that phase of treatment, Lucia had come to believe that she could function effectively on her own and that she deserved to experience emotions independent of her former boyfriend. Both Lucia and her social worker felt she was ready to move on to a new phase of therapy and consider tackling some of the secondary problems on her list, given that the acute stressor for which she had initially entered treatment was no longer pressing.

There were a number of potential domains. Lucia reported persistent hypochondriacal concerns that she had been experiencing since the age of 9, when her mother had left her family. She also reported a past history of substance abuse (both cocaine and alcohol). Although she was no longer using drugs or drinking heavily, Lucia still felt that she used alcohol to manage her emotions and did not like relying on a substance to cope. Furthermore, Lucia had many problems at work, where she felt that her boss and coworkers took advantage of her and regularly made unreasonable requests on her time. As a result, Lucia worked long hours, resented some of her coworkers, and felt disappointed in her own lack of assertiveness. Both Lucia and her social worker agreed that although she had made tremendous gains in establishing emotional independence and stability in her personal life, these new skills had not adequately generalized to her work environment.

When the clinician asked what problem area was the biggest concern to her, Lucia replied that she was sick of worrying about being ill and wanted to focus on this problem during the next phase of treatment. The therapist was surprised, because the client had only mentioned fears of illness very occasionally, yet she complained almost every session about her frustrating work situation. Rather than force her own agenda on the client, the social worker suggested that Lucia monitor both problems. Lucia agreed to rate and record her frustration levels at work (and instances of unassertive behavior, such as not saying "no" when it would have been appropriate), as well as the frequency and duration of her worries about becoming ill.

At the next session, Lucia was surprised to report that she had only thought about getting cancer a few minutes every other day. On the other hand, each workday, she had rated her frustration levels at 90 out of 100. The social worker asked whether Lucia thought this pattern was typical of other weeks, and Lucia agreed that it was. Informed by the data about the impact of different problems, Lucia and her clinician quickly agreed on a plan of action. They decided to focus on assertiveness training for the next phase of treatment, with the idea that they would continue to monitor her drinking and somatic concerns, so that they could switch the focus of treatment if these other problems escalated.

Interestingly, Lucia spontaneously decided to reduce her drinking midway through this second phase of treatment (even though this was not an explicit aim of the therapy at that time). The combination of emotion management from the first phase and assertiveness training in the second phase of therapy had provided Lucia with a much broader range of coping responses when she felt upset, whether at home or at work. Consequently, she no longer felt as compelled to drink in response to negative affect.

Lucia's social worker took a very collaborative approach to treatment planning, expecting that she and her client could agree on the aims of treatment by talking through the relevant issues and supporting their decisions with data. At the other end of the collaborative continuum are clinicians who take full responsibility for the Problem List at all phases. The information on the list often comes from the client, but there are many instances in which a fully collaborative approach is not suitable. For example, the clinician may believe the client is manipulating the Problem List for secondary gain, as in the case of a client trying to get a particular diagnosis to receive more benefits and compensation. Other clients may be too focused on blaming others for their problems to collaborate effectively, as is often the case with domestic violence offenders. In these cases, clients may remain as unaware of the Problem List as they are of other clinical documentation, such as progress notes. Even clients who never physically see the Problem List will naturally be involved in its creation. Only the client can give an indication of his or her level of motivation to work on particular problems, and this obviously will be a factor in prioritizing items on the list.

Between the wholly collaborative and completely clinician-driven models lie many alternatives that make up the middle ground in which most therapists operate. For example, the therapist may make an initial Problem List in full collaboration with the client, to be sure that all of the client's presenting concerns are included. He or she may then take a second look at the Problem List and add items without explicitly consulting the client. As we discussed earlier, these may be clinically appropriate problems that the client is not yet ready to endorse, such as excessive alcohol consumption or overdependence on a spouse. This also occurs frequently when working with children; clients may be unaware of some of the behaviors that are perceived as problematic by either their parents or the school system. The therapist may wish to monitor some problems that the client is less concerned about; the Problem List serves as a reminder in this regard.

For example, Sam was a man who sought treatment for his panic disorder. He described a workaholic lifestyle in which he felt tremendous pressure to succeed. Having already established remarkable financial success, he nevertheless felt pressure continually to top his previous achievements (and salary), in order to be seen as successful by his family and peers. Working and commuting took about 18 hours of each day, and he had maintained this lifestyle for 10 years. Sam's therapist responded to his request for treatment of panic disorder, but she also viewed his relentless drive for achievement as likely contributing to the onset of his panic and placing him at risk for future difficulties with anxiety and depression. The therapist developed the parts of the Problem List that pertained to panic in collaboration with Sam, but she also listed and monitored problems related to his drive for success without explicitly discussing them with Sam.

CASE FORMULATION AND THE PROBLEM LIST

Thus far, we have discussed the Problem List as something developed at the outset of therapy, in conjunction with the initial assessment. The Problem List can also be an integral part of case formulation. As defined by Eells (1997), case formulation is "a hypothesis about the causes, precipitants, and maintaining influences of a person's psychological, interpersonal, and behavioral problems" (p. 1). Creation of the Problem List can facilitate case formulation, because it includes problems that will not be explicitly targeted by treatment yet illuminate issues that will be addressed.

Case formulation includes information about the client as well as treatment recommendations. Although the content of some aspects of the case formulation will vary depending on the theoretical perspective of the clinician, the formulation is an orderly arrangement of data and treatment plans that follows some rational principles (Sperry, Gudeman, Blackwell, & Faulkner, 1992). Eells (1997) notes that case formulation can offer a complement to traditional diagnostic systems that use descriptive symptom subsets as a basis for classification (e.g., DSM-IV) by focusing on causes, precipitants, and maintaining influences. A richer understanding can accommodate the diverse backgrounds and problems that characterize clients in ways that a simple diagnostic label is unable to capture. Additionally, a case formulation can help reconcile and integrate information from an Axis I and Axis II assessment, such as how a client's personality style maintains or exacerbates her or his primary psychological problem.

Sperry et al. (1992) argued that well-constructed case formulations have three components in common, regardless of the theoretical orientation of the practitioner. The formulation begins with a *descriptive* component, which involves a phenomenological statement about the nature, severity, and precipitant(s) of the client's presenting problem(s). Good formulations also include an *explanatory* component, in which the clinician briefly outlines his or her understanding of the factors that led to the development and maintenance of symptoms and dysfunctional life patterns. Finally, also included, is a *treatment/prognosis* component, which is an explicit blueprint governing planned interventions and outlining the clinician's expectations for the degree and type of change that can be expected. Interested readers are referred to Turkat (1985) and Bruch and Bond (1998) for more detail on composing a case formulation.

Not only does the Problem List enhance case formulation, but also case formulation may inform and shape the Problem List. The checklist of biopsychosocial domains that we provide is meant to be a minimal list of areas to consider for inclusion on the Problem List. As the therapist develops ideas about the case conceptualization, hypotheses will arise about related problems that may also be pertinent. These hypotheses flow naturally from the case conceptualization. As the clinician continues to develop the case formulation, these hypotheses are tested by further assessment, which often reveals previously undiscovered problems to add to the list.

For example, Suejin was a client who sought treatment because she was ashamed to use public toilets for fear that people would think bad things about her if she took too much time in the stall. The therapist originally pursued a straightforward exposure-based therapy based on her conceptualization of Suejin's problem as social phobia. Over time, however, conversations with Suejin revealed material that caused the therapist to amend her case formulation to include more general issues of shame and morality related to sexuality. Because of this change in the case formulation, the therapist explicitly assessed Suejin's sexual functioning and discovered that she was anorgasmic in her sexual relationship with her husband, and that the relationship had suffered from Suejin's conflicts between her religious beliefs and sexuality. In this case, the case formulation led the therapist to ask questions about problems that would eventually be added to the Problem List. These problems, which Suejin would not have raised without direct questioning, were then addressed in a subsequent phase of treatment.

As Persons and Tompkins (1997) note, integrating case formulation and problem assessment can also help the therapist to predict obstacles to the implementation of the treatment plan. An explicit case formulation undoubtedly enhances the clinician's ability to carry out effective assessment and to efficiently develop treatment plans. In many clinical settings, the case formulation will also facilitate the writing of required formal treatment plans, discharge summaries, and justifications for further treatment. The benefits of case formulation are not limited to a specific theoretical approach, just as the development of the Problem List is a transtheoretical endeavor. We illustrate some of the interplay of the case formulation and the Problem List by introducing the case of Anna.

Anna, a 39-year-old married woman, initially presented for treatment of what she called an eating disorder. Anna complained that whenever she ate a meal, she became very short of breath (dyspnea). She felt that she could not get enough air into her lungs, and she worried that something was wrong with her. Upon further evaluation, the clinician learned that Anna placed a premium on being thin. When she began to eat a meal, she questioned whether she was hungry enough to make eating "worth it" in terms of the enjoyment she would receive from the food versus the calories she would consume. Although quite focused on her body shape and weight, Anna was of normal weight. Food records indicated adequate (although regimented) intake of calories, and she denied having binges.

Anna's description of her work revealed hints of an overly careful approach and perhaps excessive concern about evaluation. She described having trouble in her work as an accountant, because she was much more careful (and hence slower) than other accountants in her firm. She got up at 4:30 A.M. most mornings, went to the gym daily, worked very long hours, and arrived home in time to have a quick bite of supper before falling into bed. Anna was not satisfied with her job and felt constantly on edge, because she feared she might be caught making a mistake. She had long ago given up hope of becoming a partner in the firm.

After the clinician elicited these descriptive details about Anna's problem, she then began to think about the explanatory component of the formulation, which led to further evaluation. Anna clearly described the development of dyspnea during meals as the precipitant that caused her to seek treatment, and the therapist viewed this as a reflection of the anxiety Anna experienced due to her conflict between the need to eat and her concern about body shape and weight. These integrative details would not necessarily have been revealed had the therapist relied solely on a DSM-IV classification of Anna's problems. Explicitly listing Anna's problems provided the therapist with a concise overview of all the problems. The Problem List served as a visual tool to help the therapist work through a case formulation, conduct additional assessment, and prioritize the target problems for treatment.

In considering possible factors that may have influenced the development of her intense concern with her weight, the therapist first considered Anna's family relationships. Anna was adopted at the age of 2, after the suicide of her biological mother. Her relationship with her adoptive mother appeared to contribute to her focus on body shape and weight. Anna's adoptive mother frequently voiced her high expectations for Anna. She referred to Anna's education in elite private schools as a basis for her high expectations, and Anna had come to feel that she needed to achieve extraordinary career success just to be considered "average" given her education. Furthermore, Anna's mother ridiculed members of the family who were overweight, berating them when they were not present. Anna's mother overtly monitored the body weight of everyone in the family, even asking Anna how much her sister weighed.

The therapist also observed that Anna's perfectionistic style appeared to contribute to her concern about her shape and weight, as well as the problems she described at work. The therapist began to formulate hypotheses about how aspects of Anna's personality style may impact on other areas of functioning. Upon inquiry, it became clear that Anna's perfectionism also caused problems in her marriage, because she had exceptionally high standards for cleanliness at home. For example, she changed and washed the sheets on her bed every other evening when she came home from work rather than waiting until the weekend, when she had more time. When Anna's husband insisted that she allow him to do some of the housecleaning, Anna permitted him to do so but then criticized his work. At times she would redo things, such as refolding the laundry if her husband did not follow her strict standards.

These interpersonal problems were included on the Problem List when they became apparent as the therapist developed her case formulation. See Figure 2.3 for Anna's initial Problem List. The first six items were added to the Problem List on the basis of the initial evaluation. (Note that Anna did not endorse her regimented eating or exercise patterns as problematic, because she viewed them as necessary strategies to control her weight.) The remaining items were added as the therapist developed her understanding of the factors that provoked and maintained Anna's presenting problem.

	Client endorsed?
1. Dyspnea when eating	√
2. Eats supper very late	√
3. Regimented eating pattern	
4. Regimented exercise habits	
5. Dissatisfaction with job	√
6. Pressure and criticism from mother	√
7. Disagreements with husband over household tasks	
8. Extremely high standards for tasks related to work	
9. Overly concerned about appearances	

FIGURE 2.3. Problem List for Anna: Informed by case formulation.

PRIORITIZING PROBLEMS

Once the initial evaluation and case formulation are complete, the therapist goes back to the Problem List and checks to be sure that all of the important areas implicated in the case formulation are addressed. It is rarely feasible to work on all of a client's problems at once, so the next step in treatment planning is to prioritize the problems that require immediate attention and determine which ones can wait. Chapter 3 describes the process of formulating treatment aims for the first (and subsequent) phase of therapy, but we briefly touch on the issue of prioritizing items on the Problem List here.

As can be seen from the examples given in this chapter, the Problem List is likely to be quite long for many clients. We have listed the items on each list in the order in which we learned about them from the client, rather than in a prioritized order, because this is how our own Problem Lists look in practice. For clients who face serious and complicated problems, the Problem List quickly becomes lengthy and unwieldy. As most seasoned practitioners know, a number of factors influence the relative priority each problem takes in treatment planning. Some of the pertinent considerations include (1) the client's agreement in acknowledging a problem, (2) the case formulation, (3) the impact of each problem on the client's functioning, (4) the impact of each problem on significant others, (5) the probability of success in tackling each problem (especially with respect to the amount of time the client has for treatment), (6) the client's readiness or motivation to change a particular behavior, (7) the likelihood of improvement on one problem generalizing to another problem area, and (8) the degree to which other caregivers are also involved in the case. In the next few pages, we discuss some of these points in more detail.

Using the Case Formulation to Prioritize Problems

As discussed earlier, the case formulation represents the clinician's educated hypothesis about how the client's various problems fit together and are maintained. Usually, this formulation will also generate ideas about which problems are key targets for a broader resolution of the client's difficulties. For example, socially anxious and avoidant behavior in several different settings may be secondary to a client's difficulty engaging in assertive behavior, so targeting assertive behavior may result in a positive domino effect. In addition, the formulation often incorporates the therapist's ideas about aspects of the client's style or situation that are likely to facilitate or interfere with treatment. For instance, a client who expresses ambivalence about changing a problem behavior, such as reducing or quitting smoking, may require an initial intervention to increase motivation to change. Thus, the case formulation usually implies a prioritization of some problems over others in terms of the order in which they should be addressed.

Impact on Functioning

Therapists usually place a higher priority on those problems that present the biggest obstacles to the client's social, occupational, and familial functioning. In the case of Francine, frequent absences from work were obviously the most disruptive problem on her list. Calling in sick on a regular basis significantly reduced her income and led to an unstable work history. Furthermore, Francine reported that her problems with work were an additional strike against her in the custody battle with her ex-husband. The therapist accordingly viewed this as a high-priority problem, because it impacted on Francine's functioning in several ways; it contributed to other problems, and resolving the problems at work could help to improve Francine's feelings of self-worth.

Impact on Family Members

Family members may receive more or less consideration in the prioritization of his or her problems, depending on the age of the client and the nature of the client's problems. Clients who are dependent on family members, such as children, those with disabilities, and the elderly, are often brought to treatment when their problems become overly disruptive to the rest of the family. In these cases, clinicians tend to place a high priority on problems that impact the family. That said, the impact on family members may also be a factor in prioritization of problems in less obvious ways. For example, her therapist was concerned about the impact of Francine's behavior on her daughters, particularly in terms of Francine's inconsistent parenting style. Although Francine did not seem especially troubled by her parenting style at the time she sought treatment, the therapist believed that helping Francine to improve her relationship with her daughters would also improve the way Francine saw herself as a person. Assessing a problem's impact on the family may not only aid in prioritizing the problem but also may inform particular treatment procedures. For example, a family intervention may be indicated when a child's temper tantrums are made worse by the response from parents and siblings.

Probability of Success

All else being equal, problems that are believed to have a good prognosis are often addressed earlier in treatment. Obviously, this does not mean that the therapist will place a higher priority on noncentral problems or problems not associated with functional impairment. However, within the realm of problems that share similar levels of urgency and centrality to the case formulation, therapists often choose to begin with those problems that are likely to show relatively quick progress.

For example, several of the items on Francine's Problem List involved symptoms of depression, including sadness, anxiety, fatigue, insomnia, weight gain, and feeling worthless. Some of these items would be prioritized higher than others, because of their connection to Francine's occupational impairment. For instance, the therapist may believe that helping Francine to regulate her sleeping habits would improve her insomnia and reduce her fatigue within a brief time, so these problems may be addressed ahead of others.

One of the benefits of working on relatively malleable problems early in treatment is that it may boost the client's motivation for treatment and hopefulness about the likelihood of success. Early improvement, even on a relatively small issue, can help clients feel ready to make changes, because they now have tangible experience with a payoff as a result of making changes in their life patterns. Furthermore, having a small success and seeing positive changes may help clients to loosen resistance about addressing more challenging problems. Bandura (1977) has discussed how creating a sense of efficacy and mastery can lead to broader, more enduring behavior change (which we describe in greater detail in Chapter 3).

Other Caregivers

In many settings, only one clinician will have contact with a client during any given episode of care. Clients with more serious mental health problems, however, often require multidisciplinary teams of caregivers, including psychiatrists, social workers, nutritionists, physical therapists, and others. Each of these professionals will have a unique background and training, and is likely to conceptualize the client's problems quite differently. These differences are the primary value of a multidisciplinary team, because clients seen in such settings have problems that require a complicated treatment plan. However, in practical terms, members of the treatment team will often take primary responsibility for a specific subset of the items on the Problem List, or they may formulate separate Problem Lists as appropriate for their disciplines.

Each caregiver in such a setting must take into account the bigger picture of the treatment team when prioritizing problems for a treatment plan. Even in settings that do not typically involve multidisciplinary teams, similar issues may arise. For example, the client may be referred to a specialist for some aspect of treatment, although the main responsibility for treatment rests with the generalist clinician. For example, one schizophrenic client, whose primary caregivers were a multidisciplinary team in the local community mental health center, was referred to us for brief specialty treatment of his panic attacks (precipitated by some of his psychotic symptoms).

Discussing how to prioritize problems within a multidisciplinary treatment setting (e.g., home-based care) can also highlight opportunities for collaboration. For example, an older adult at risk for a stroke or transient ischemic attack may have difficulty complying with a high blood pressure medication regimen, because he cannot remember to take his medicine. Defining this as a high priority problem may lead to clear assessment (e.g., neuropsychological evaluation of memory and cognitive functioning) and treatment roles (e.g., memory and compliance interventions) for members of the multidisciplinary team.

REEXAMINING THE PROBLEM LIST

Up to this point, we have discussed the Problem List as a task that the therapist undertakes primarily at the beginning of treatment. The bulk of the list may be constructed in collaboration with the client during the initial evaluation, and the therapist may add items as she or he develops a case formulation. However, the Problem List needs continual reexamination. With proper tending, it can aid the therapist in ongoing treatment planning. In this section, we discuss some of the conditions that motivate clinicians to reconsider the Problem List, as well as some of the benefits of maintaining an up-to-date Problem List.

New Problems Arise

We rely on the Problem List to keep track of all of the client's problems, large and small, that are the focus of treatment or not, and under the client's influence or not. This level of organization may not be as important for a new trainee with only one or two cases, but for the busy professional with dozens of cases, the Problem List can provide a quick review of not only the client's presenting problems but also some elements of the context and challenging factors in the client's environment. In order for this to be useful, the Problem List obviously needs to be kept up-to-date.

Clients may raise new problems in several different ways. Probably the most common way that clinicians learn about new problems is when clients share more detail about themselves and their presenting problems. Some types of problems are inherently shameful for clients, such as substance abuse, certain types of obsessive ideation, binge eating, child abuse, and many others. Clients often feel uncomfortable talking about problems of an intimate nature (e.g., sexual functioning), and they often begin to reveal more information about these problems as they develop a more trusting relationship with the therapist. In addition to old problems that come to light as the alliance develops, new problems may also develop as a result of life events.

Anna, whom we described earlier in the chapter, raised new problems in both of these ways. As she became more comfortable with the therapist, she began to share more information about her ritualized eating habits. She also consented to have her husband to speak to the therapist, and he contributed new observations that Anna had been reluctant to describe, such as the fact that she had begun teaching daily, aerobics classes in addition to her usual daily running routine. This new information helped the therapist to list more detailed aspects of Anna's presenting problem. In the midst of therapy, however, Anna's husband lost his job. This development did not present a financial crisis, because they were well off financially, but it did raise some problems relevant to Anna's concern about appearances, so the therapist added it to her list.

Other new problems may arise when the client begins to endorse something that he or she has not previously endorsed. For example, recall that Francine initially reported that she had no current romantic relationship. She had described dating as something she would like to do but that was low on her priority list compared to her other problems. After several months, an issue arose that made it clear that Francine was involved in a relationship with a married man in another state, whom she had met on the Internet. Although Francine maintained that they had never met in person, the relationship was clearly adding to her difficulties, because the man's wife was seeking a divorce, based in part on his relationship with Francine. Francine spent quite a bit of time with this man, conversing by phone and by computer. The therapist conceptualized this as a problem for Francine because she invested a lot of time and negative emotional energy (e.g., worrying about his divorce) in this relationship, without receiving the benefits she sought from a romantic relationship, such as companionship, physical intimacy, and a sense of partnership. After discussing these issues, Francine's therapist added several new problems to her Problem List.

New problems sometimes arise in treatment as a result of a crisis. When clients raise new issues that are distressing to them, therapists have to make relatively quick decisions about how to incorporate the new problems with others that are the focus of treatment. The Problem List can be a helpful tool in this regard, particularly if it is used collaboratively. Some clients raise crisis issues relatively often, as illustrated by the case of Kelly in Chapter 1, which can derail treatment planning if they come to control the content and direction of sessions. After hearing a client describe an emergent problem, a therapist who has been using the Problem List collaboratively can bring out the list and work with the client on adding the new problem to the list. The therapist and client can then make decisions together about how this new problem fits with other problems and whether it is important enough that the focus of treatment should be shifted from the previous treatment focus to the new problem.

Although this occurs relatively rarely, new problems can also arise following from the changes a person has made in treatment. For example, Geneva had struggled with severe obsessive–compulsive disorder (OCD) for the previous 15 years. She was essentially housebound, because the vast majority of her day was consumed by cleaning rituals. Consequently, her husband had taken on the brunt of managing the house as well as caring for their 10-year-old twins. After 4 months in therapy, Geneva's time spent conducting rituals had been cut nearly in half and her mobility was greatly increased.

Geneva now wanted to take more responsibility for child care and gain control of the family finances. This created conflict between Geneva and her husband, because it required a shift in the family power structure. Geneva had always been the "sick one" that her husband took care of, and her new independence led to a reorganization of family responsibilities and necessitated decisions about how to jointly raise their children. The therapist added marital conflict to the Problem List but, based on the feedback from both Geneva and her husband (who despite their fighting were extremely happy about the reduction of OCD symptoms), decided to continue to focus solely on the OCD in treatment before addressing the new family issues.

By putting an emergent problem on the Problem List, the client can feel reassured that the therapist has noted the problem and attended to its importance even if the focus of the session then returns to the original agenda. Going through the process of reviewing and prioritizing new problems in light of more long-standing ones can also help those clients who need to develop similar skills in managing issues that arise in daily living. Some clients feel overwhelmed by the issues facing them, and one strategy to help them feel more in control is to focus on the highest priority task. Prioritizing the Problem List can also help to reduce feelings of anxiety that new therapists may experience when inundated with a long list of serious problems. At times, crises and less serious new problems will indeed represent the highest priority; reviewing the Problem List can help both client and therapist evaluate whether this is the case.

New Phases of Treatment

Even when new problems do not arise, the therapist (and client, if working collaboratively) will want to review the Problem List each time treatment moves into a new phase. What we mean by "phases" of treatment will become clearer in the next chapter, but for now we note that treatment planning is often conducted in discrete phases, as the therapist focuses on one set of problems at a time. When the therapist decides to focus on a different set of problems (ideally, due to improvement in the first set, but not always for this reason), he or she will need to revisit the Problem List to organize new treatment aims, as well as treatment and measurement strategies.

Reviewing the Problem List with the client can provide a useful opportunity to check on the therapist's understanding of the client's problems from the initial evaluation. The client's perspective on the problems may have changed somewhat due to the effect of time or some aspect of the earlier phase of treatment. Furthermore, some problems may not seem as urgent as they once did. Asking explicitly about each problem allows the clinician greater confidence that she or he is making judgments with an accurate understanding of the client's concerns.

In some settings, clients typically come for a single course of therapy. Whether the treatment lasts a single session or several years, the clinician does not expect to see the client again once treatment ends. In other settings, however, due to the payment structure or the types of problems experienced by the clientele, therapists can expect to see clients repeatedly as they enter therapy for a relatively brief episode of treatment, stop therapy, and then return at another point for another episode of care. The therapist can begin a new episode of treatment by reviewing the Problem List from the last episode, crossing off items that are no longer relevant and adding new ones. The Problem List can thus contribute to continuity of care in a relatively efficient way.

For example, Harold was a 60-year-old, single man with recurrent major depression and OCD. He was also partially blind (having only peripheral vision), and many of his obsessions and compulsions revolved around cleaning and maintaining his custom-made glasses. Harold had been in and out of treatment settings over the past 20 years, and each time he sought treatment, his practitioners had to go through the process of "catching up" on the status of Harold's problems. The benefits of creating a formalized Problem List were clear to Harold's treaters. First of all, Harold's past patterns indicated that he was likely to be in treatment for a relatively short period of time (until his depressive symptoms stabilized). However, he was very likely to return to treatment at a later date, when his depressive symptoms returned.

The Problem List offered an easy starting-point for Harold's treaters. Using the Problem List developed during Harold's last depressive episode, his treaters were quickly and easily reminded of Harold's more predictable problems, such as his poor sleeping habits, social isolation that typically accompanied his depression, and his rituals surrounding his glasses. Nevertheless, Harold's Problem List was not static. For many years, Harold had held a steady job but had no romantic relationship. When he sought treatment most recently, however, Harold had lost his job but was involved in his first ongoing romance and was considering having his "woman friend" move in with him. Problems related to these life changes were added to Harold's Problem List. This proved beneficial not only for Harold's treaters, but also for Harold, who appreciated having a list to refer back to, noting that it was reassuring and indicative of the extent to which his treaters attended to him. Being able to cross items off his list also gave Harold a sense that he was making some progress despite his repeated need for episodes of care.

SHORTCUTS FOR THE BUSY CLINICIAN

The Problem List is probably one of the easiest components of the PACC approach to implement, because it is most likely to be a part of routine practice already. However, we have found some strategies that can help make this list an especially useful tool for treatment planning. The process of comprehensively surveying a client's problems, selecting the issues most in need of urgent care, and continually reexamining the list of problems reflects our belief that therapy is a flexible and dynamic challenge. We offer the following suggestions to make the Problem List work most efficiently, in the hopes that they will be helpful, particularly for beginning therapists who have not yet developed their assessment style.

1. *Develop the Problem List collaboratively with the client in session during the assessment phase.* Have an blank copy of the Problem List handy and jot notes on it as the initial assessment proceeds, rather than writing freeform notes and formulating the Problem List later. As you develop ideas about the case formulation, use this opportunity to evaluate potential issues related to the presenting problem. Completing the list in session reduces the likelihood that a problem will be forgotten or not recorded, and it demonstrates to the client that his or her problems are being heard and taken seriously.

2. *Use the checklist of biopsychosocial problem areas during the assessment interview.* Keep a copy of the checklist nearby as you do the initial assessment, as a reminder of problem areas about which you want to inquire. Covering all the important domains will facilitate the process of case formulation and treatment planning.

3. *Modify the Problem List format to better align with required clinical documentation in your setting.* If your organization already has a form for listing or prioritizing the client's problems, use it! Some of the forms clinicians complete are purely administrative, with little value for the actual treatment. The Problem List is one form that can be constructive, so feel free to bend the recommended procedures to fit them to your setting. The main objective is to develop and carefully monitor a comprehensive Problem List; the format of the list is less important.

CHAPTER 3

TREATMENT PLANNING USING A PHASE APPROACH

Treatment planning involves mapping not only the direction taken to meet the needs of the clients but also the tools used along the way. Planning also involves formulating expectations about how much change is anticipated and how quickly it should occur. A number of clinicians have emphasized the importance of treatment planning (e.g., Galasso, 1987; Makover, 1992, 1996), and these days many managed care organizations require it. As Heinssen, Levendusky, and Hunter (1995) described, "Focused, well-articulated treatment plans [improve] communication with managed care agencies because each client's presenting problems, treatment goals, and interventions are specified in understandable terms" (p. 530). Contemporary mental health care providers are usually bound by significant time constraints, so they must focus treatment strategies to accomplish as much as possible in just a few sessions. Given these constraints, treatment planning is a necessary element of accountable practice. Creating a Treatment Plan can help to organize a client's problems into a set of measurable goals and intervention strategies that maximize the efficiency of practice.

Nonetheless, treatment planning may be difficult for some practitioners to embrace, perhaps because it appears to be incompatible with the artistry and spontaneity that attract many individuals to the practice of psychotherapy. Makover (1996), who noted that an "anti-planning bias" has permeated the culture of psychotherapy over the years, argued for setting aside this bias, in part because it is based on three questionable assumptions: (1) human behavior is mysterious and unpredictable; (2) humans are too complex to be subject to rational planning; and (3) the relationship in psychotherapy is more important than the therapeutic activity. Makover suggests instead (and we agree) that psychotherapy is understandable, teachable, and amenable to a planning process. Although human behavior is complex and often un-predictable, contemporary practice of clinical psychology, clinical so-cial work, and psychiatry involves identifiable therapeutic strategies that can be specified or sketched out in advance. A positive therapeutic alliance appears to be necessary for good therapy outcomes, but it is not the only critical element (Bergin & Garfield, 1994).

FROM PROBLEM IDENTIFICATION TO PROBLEM SOLVING

Once the Problem List is created (as detailed in Chapter 2), the thera-pist moves from problem identification to problem solving, an iterative process in the PACC model. After cataloguing the client's problems, the therapist specifies aims that represent short-term goals related to the most pressing problems and are targets of the initial stage of inter-vention. The therapist then outlines treatment strategies to achieve these aims, measures how effectively the client is progressing toward them, and regularly reviews progress to determine whether the treat-ment should change, remain the same, or end. In short, treatment plan-ning is a systematic way to move through the Problem List.

TREATMENT PLANNING AS THE THERAPIST'S MAP

Of course, it is impossible to address all of the client's problems at once. In our own practices, we weigh the options, often in collabora-tion with the client, to come up with a tentative "map" of the treat-ment process—essentially a brief plan of priorities and interventions. The challenge for the therapist is to synthesize the data that have been gathered from the initial interview and to formulate a case con-ceptualization that targets the treatment to the particular problems and strengths of the client. As we have discussed in Chapters 1 and 2, the therapist need not be constrained by a single therapeutic orientation, but can instead use an integrative approach that flexibly adapts the initial Treatment Plan based on the client's response to the intervention. By combining an evidence-based approach to selection of treatment strategies with ongoing measurement of progress, the therapist can avoid falling into the trap of offering all clients the same treatment, regardless of the nature of their difficulties (see Lewis & Usdin, 1982).

The case formulation bridges the Problem List and the Treatment Plan, acting as "the clinician's compass" (Sperry et al., 1992) to guide treatment. As discussed in Chapter 2, effective case formulation includes descriptive components ("What is happening to the client?"), explanatory components ("Why did it happen?"), and treatment–prognostic components ("What can be done, and how effective is it likely to be?"; Sperry et al., 1992). Whereas the formulation is the therapist's compass, the Treatment Plan is the map, detailing where the therapy is headed and likely paths to reach the destination. The therapist uses the case formulation's descriptive, explanatory, and treatment–prognostic components to help integrate the biological, psychological, and social underpinnings of the client's difficulties. This groundwork informs the order in which problems are best addressed, the expectations for change, and the treatments that are most likely to be helpful (Lewis & Usdin, 1982).

For example, a client who is dissatisfied with her marriage may seek treatment for a number of reasons. Understanding why she is dissatisfied is not only the explanatory component of the case formulation, but it also influences the therapist's selection of interventions and his or her expectations for treatment. If the client's marital dissatisfaction is grounded in her belief that she is unlovable, the therapist is likely to choose initial interventions to address such beliefs. On the other hand, if the dissatisfaction appears to be due to the client's lack of identity outside of marriage, the therapist is likely to choose different interventions. If the dissatisfaction comes from the client's inability to be assertive and to communicate effectively with her spouse, the interventions will be different still. The degree to which the client is coming to treatment to "fix" the marriage versus "escape" it is also a part of the formulation that helps to dictate expectations for change. If the client comes from a background in which divorce is common or accepted, the expectations may be slightly different than if she believes that divorce is unacceptable. There is no right or wrong answer to how the formulation should guide treatment planning, and different clinicians have their own preferences as to where to begin an intervention.

Nonetheless, the formulation helps therapists to prioritize goals and create plans for change.

Realistic Goal Setting

Task performance is greatly enhanced by setting goals related to the task. This is one of the most robust and replicable findings in psychology (Locke, Shaw, Saari, & Latham, 1981). A client who works toward a goal is more likely to make productive use of the therapy sessions and of the time between sessions. Furthermore, goal setting enhances the tendency of the client to persist in the face of inevitable obstacles, and focusing on the goals encourages the client and therapist to develop creative strategies to attain the goal.

An important factor influencing the type of goals set is the client's efficacy expectations. As Bandura (1977) described, an *outcome expectation* is a person's belief that certain behaviors will lead to certain outcomes (e.g., "Exercise will improve my mood and make me feel good about myself"). An *efficacy expectation* is the person's belief that he or she will successfully carry out the behavior (e.g., "I can meet my goal of exercising three times a week"). Often, the client may expect good outcomes but have low confidence in his or her ability to carry out the planned changes. For example, "I know spending time with my friends will make me feel better, but I simply can't bring myself to pick up that phone and dial." Efficacy expectations are critical because the strength of clients' convictions in their own effectiveness is likely to affect whether they will even try new strategies for coping with their problems (Bandura, 1977). As a consequence, even therapists who use a very collaborative style may need to take the lead in setting goals if a client is demoralized because of low efficacy expectations.

Goal Acceptance and Commitment

Motivation to establish goals in psychotherapy comes from within the client as well as from external sources (e.g., family, therapists, agencies). Nevertheless, even the most agreeable and motivated clients may have difficulty maintaining commitment to established goals. (Indeed, this is often part of the problem that brings clients to treatment.) As therapists, how can we help boost clients' motivation and commitment to achieving therapy-related goals? Setting concrete goals that are challenging yet realistic is one way to help make this happen (Locke et al., 1981). Encouraging clients to make a public commitment to the goal also increases goal commitment (Hollenbeck, Williams, & Klein, 1989). The simple act of discussing treatment aims with a therapist (or with other members of a treatment group) can function as a public commitment, or clients can go further and discuss goals with trusted friends or family members. We recommend looking into motivational interviewing (Miller & Rollnick, 1991) for specific strategies to evaluate and enhance commitment to change for those clients who need a motivational boost.

TREATMENT PHASES

The PACC approach views treatment as a series of phases rather than as a single overall target or intervention. In general, it is only possible to work on a limited number of problems at once. Some clients with relatively straightforward and circumscribed problems may need only one phase of therapy, but more complicated clients will progress through several phases. Within each phase, the therapist (usually in collaboration with the client) defines aims that are to be the focus of that particular section of therapy, develops a measurement plan for those aims, and specifies the intervention strategies to be used within the phase. See Figure 3.1 for a blank copy of the form we use for this aspect of treatment planning.

The client should be included in the decision-making process to determine where to focus treatment initially. Consider the case of Peter, a 15-year-old high school sophomore, who had been experiencing panic attacks for the past year. Peter had been taking antianxiety medication prescribed by his primary care physician who was a family friend. In March of his sophomore year, Peter's panic attacks became so severe that he was spending every day in the nurse's office rather than attending his classes. His guidance counselors became increasingly concerned, and Peter began to feel isolated and hopeless about his condition. In April, he took an overdose of Tylenol and was hospitalized. Although his parents were reluctant to acknowledge that Peter had emotional problems, they nevertheless enrolled him in a short-term residential treatment program for adolescents. During this therapy, Peter revealed that he not only experienced panic attacks but also had a fear of vomiting that prohibited him from eating regular, balanced meals. In the 2 months leading up to his hospitalization, Peter had lost over 20% of his body weight, putting him at risk for multiple health problems.

Peter's problems crossed multiple domains of concern, including his depression and suicide attempt, panic attacks, agoraphobia, fear of vomiting, severe weight loss, and his parents' tendency to minimize his problems (which could undermine treatment progress). Not all of Peter's problems could be addressed at once. Instead, using a phase model, the treatment team at the residential program worked with Peter and his family to create a plan of action. Obviously, the high-risk problems, including Peter's suicidality, had to be addressed before his other problems could be tackled in subsequent phases of treatment. Conceptualizing treatment in terms of phases requires a degree of patience and an open acknowledgment to the client (and in Peter's case, to his parents) that not everything will get better at once.

The assumption that therapy can only target a limited number of problems at one time means that the "current" aims of treatment will shift over time. In Peter's case, the initial treatment aims were to minimize suicide risk and improve his depressed mood. Once Peter's mood was stabilized, the treatment aims changed. Although there were a number of possible problem areas to target (e.g., family relationships, panic attacks, weight loss through food avoidance), the therapist and Peter chose to focus on his panic attacks and avoidance of school. This issue was a priority for Peter because summer school had begun and, having been a high-achieving student, Peter wanted to begin making up the work he had missed due to his illness. Simultaneously, Peter's therapist arranged for a consultation with a nutritionist to partially address his weight loss. In this way, Peter worked on multiple problems concurrently without detracting from the focus on his panic. See Figure 3.2 to see how Peter's therapist completed the Aims portion of the Treatment Plan for the first two phases of therapy.

The number of phases clients will need depends on several factors, including the number and severity of their problems. Some clients come to therapy to work on a discrete problem, such as a specific phobia. Others come to treatment with multiple, complicated problems, such as a first psychotic break within the context of ongoing substance abuse, job loss, and an unsupportive home environment. Still other clients come to treatment in the midst of a depressive episode, and the true extent of their problems may not be apparent until some of the depressive symptoms subside. In contemporary models of treatment delivery, it is likely that one clinician will not be responsible for delivering all phases of care to a client. In Peter's case, for example, his primary clinician was a psychologist, but he also had sessions with a nutritionist as well as some family sessions with a social worker.

Treatment Phase I	Date:
Aims:	1.
	2.
	3.
Measures: (attach graph)	1.
	2.
	3.
Strategies:	1.
	2.
	3.

Date for Phase I Progress Review:

Treatment Phase II	Date:
Aims:	1.
	2.
	3.
Measures: (attach graph)	1.
	2.
	3.
Strategies:	1.
	2.
	3.

Date for Phase II Progress Review:

(continued)

FIGURE 3.1. Treatment Planning Worksheet.

Treatment Phase III   Date:

Aims: **1.** _____

             2. _____

             3. _____

Measures: **1.** _____
(attach
graph)   **2.** _____

             3. _____

Strategies: **1.** _____

             2. _____

             3. _____

Date for Phase III Progress Review:

Treatment Phase IV   Date:

Aims: **1.** _____

             2. _____

             3. _____

Measures: **1.** _____
(attach
graph)   **2.** _____

             3. _____

Strategies: **1.** _____

             2. _____

             3. _____

Date for Phase IV Progress Review:

FIGURE 3.1. *(continued)*

Treatment Phase I   Date: April 17, 2002

Aims: **1.** Reduce frequency of suicidal ideation.

          2. Reduce hopelessness.

          3. Reduce level of depression.

Measures: **1.**
(attach graph)
           2.

           3.

Strategies: **1.**

           2.

           3.

Date for Phase I Progress Review: June 21, 2002

Treatment Phase II   Date: June 23, 2002

Aims: **1.** Reduce frequency of panic attacks.

          2. Reduce fear of having more attacks.

          3. Eliminate avoidance of school and social situations.

Measures: **1.**
(attach graph)
           2.

           3.

Strategies: **1.**

           2.

           3.

Date for Phase II Progress Review: September 25, 2002

FIGURE 3.2. Aims of Phase I and II Treatment Plan for Peter.

EFFECTIVENESS OF PHASE MODELS OF PSYCHOTHERAPY

Rogers (1958) was among the first clinicians to describe distinct phases of psychotherapy, noting an early phase in which clients struggle to identify problems, and a later phase in which clients feel a heightened sense of self-awareness and confidence. Although the specific objectives of each phase of treatment may depend upon the clinician's background and training, the notion that psychotherapy proceeds in stages is a common heuristic tool that transcends theoretical orientation (Beitman, Goldfried, & Norcross, 1989). Empirical evidence corroborates the belief that repeated "doses" of brief therapy have the same or better effect as a time-unlimited, single phase of therapy, even when treating severe and chronic conditions (Budman & Gurman, 1988). In contemporary mental health care, multiple doses (i.e., phases) of treatment are also frequently a practical reality (Haas & Cummings, 1991) due to the unavailability of sustained long-term care.

Experienced therapists often develop their own implicit system for thinking through the anticipated phases of treatment with different clients. In carrying out the PACC approach, we encourage clinicians to make this process explicit. For example, Heinssen et al. (1995) have developed a therapeutic contracting model that is compatible with ours, in which they propose a series of treatment phases with specified aims (i.e., short-term goals) and strategies. Data evaluating the effectiveness of their contracting program suggest that, across treatment settings (e.g., private and public psychiatric hospitals, outpatient settings), the program enhances treatment compliance, achieves positive therapeutic outcomes, and provides long-term, cost-effective, multimodal treatment. See Heinssen et al. (1995) for a review.

Conceptualizing treatment as consisting of distinct phases can also be useful in the treatment of Axis II disorders, even borderline personality disorder. Zanarini and Frankenburg (1994) proposed three separate phases based on their interpretation of theoretical work by writers such as Gunderson (1984), Masterson (1972), and Volkman (1987). The first phase is called "Reframing" and involves treatment strategies such as teaching clients to reframe their complaints and actions (e.g., suicidal gestures) as efforts to express intense psychological pain. Zanarini and Frankenburg (1994) argue that by the end of the first phase of treatment, one should see a decrease in the client's reliance on self-destructive behaviors and complaints, an increase in the ability to articulate the pain he or she is feeling, and an increase in his or her goal-directed activity (as indicated by a return to work or school).

In the second phase of treatment, "Validation," treatment strategies include helping clients to verbalize chaotic life experiences and allowing them to accept their emotional responses to these experiences. In the "Mourning" phase of treatment, Zanarini and Frankenburg (1994) suggest strategies that include helping clients experience and tolerate emotions (such as sorrow) associated with how others have hurt them and how they have hurt themselves and others. This model illustrates the feasibility of effectively planning therapy even for complex, long-standing problems by specifying the expected concrete changes for each phase of treatment.

The PACC approach is intended to be adaptable, enabling movement from one therapy phase to another to allow treatment to be tailored to the individual client based on his or her progress. Thus, the initial Treatment Plan is not an end product but is instead an iterative, dynamic agenda. Although many therapists will be able to foreshadow future treatment phases, there is also flexibility inherent in a phase model to accommodate the inevitable "surprises" that arise in psychotherapy. By moving the client from one phase to the next, the therapist is able to respond to unforeseen challenges and adjust to a client's changing needs, rather than adhering to a rigid approach or feeling that treatment has been derailed. We now describe our conceptualization of phases within the PACC approach.

PHASES IN THE PACC APPROACH

Each phase of treatment within the PACC approach addresses three distinct components of treatment planning: Aims, Measures, and Strategies (see Figure 3.1). We discuss treatment aims and strategies in this chapter and then describe measurement issues in Chapter 4. Briefly, aims are the short-term, specific goals set at the beginning of a treatment phase. The client and therapist may also discuss long-term, abstract treatment goals (e.g., improve life satisfaction), but these are different from treatment aims. The aims are concrete and measurable objectives that usually vary from one phase of treatment to the next. Taken as a whole, aims can be thought of as the components that contribute to an overarching treatment goal. Treatment strategies are the means by which the therapist goes about helping the client to reach the aims. In other words, strategies are the specific interventions and techniques used within the therapy session. Measures are the tools (some standardized and others tailored for a given client) that assess how much progress is being made toward a treatment aim.

These components are illustrated in the Treatment Plan for Marjorie, a 57-year-old woman who sought treatment for depression that had begun 8 years earlier, following the death of her son. Marjorie was socially isolated and lonely, and she had lost interest in most things. She had also struggled with hypothyroidism, which was being successfully managed with medication at the time she began psychotherapy. Nevertheless, she had gained about 60 pounds in the previous few years, which only deepened her sense of demoralization. Marjorie's primary goal was to stop feeling so depressed, and she also hoped to return to her former weight.

In the first phase of treatment, the therapist proposed aims that would be manageable for Marjorie and provide some momentum built on success. These aims included increasing Marjorie's social activity level, beginning a program of walking (which Marjorie said she used to enjoy), and learning to keep a diary of her automatic thoughts. Although these aims may seem modest, Marjorie's long-standing depression made them feel challenging, and Marjorie initially viewed them as weak substitutes for her real goal of feeling less depressed. Nevertheless, when the therapist explained the rationale of the Treatment Plan (that achieving these small aims would contribute to progress on her larger goal), Marjorie responded positively to having her problems broken down into manageable parts that would be addressed one by one.

OUTLINING EXPECTATIONS FOR PROGRESS WITHIN PHASES

In planning each phase of treatment, we have found it helpful to schedule an actual date for review of progress on the aims of that phase. The review date reflects the therapist's expectations about the rate at which change ought to occur relative to the specific aims in a given phase. Depending on the nature of aims in a given phase of treatment, we generally schedule Progress Reviews at least every 3 months. (See Chapter 6 for a discussion of factors affecting this flexible time line.) If the therapist does not expect change to occur in that time, then the aims should be honed to represent smaller steps of progress. Measurement of progress occurs regularly and is not limited to review dates. In this way, measurement data can be used in treatment planning both for the next phase and for specific strategies within each session. Bernstein (1992) eloquently describes the rationale for this kind of continuous Progress Review:

One might fear that a competency-based approach to therapy would present extra difficulty in cases where the client fails to progress in treatment. The opposite is true. With a competency-based approach to treatment, the structure of the therapeutic process forces both client and therapist to recognize a failure when it has occurred, rather than dodge the issue. This is tremendously helpful because with recognition there is an opportunity for corrective action and new learning. Rarely does learning occur without failure, and therefore, there is rarely successful therapy without failure. (pp. 272–273)

During the review, the therapist examines the degree to which the aims of the preceding phase have been met (based on the data collected over time during the phase). He or she then decides what to do for the next phase. A new phase may represent moving on to new aims when the current aims are accomplished, changing the strategies used, or switching to a problem that has become more pressing than the one targeted in the previous phase.

Returning to the example of Marjorie, the therapist reviewed progress on the aims of the initial phase of treatment after five sessions of therapy. Marjorie's depression had diminished somewhat, with Beck Depression Inventory scores moving from 26 to 22, but she was still quite depressed. Although initially resistant, she had begun taking 20-minute walks around her neighborhood about three times a week. Furthermore, although her social network had dwindled during her years of depression and social isolation, Marjorie had begun to strike up conversations with colleagues, neighbors, and strangers. She rediscovered that talking to people could be enjoyable. At the fifth session, her diary of social interactions showed that she was having about one social conversation each day, a vast improvement over the initial evaluation. The therapist, satisfied with the initial progress in helping Marjorie to get activated, moved on to a new phase of treatment, developing aims related to Marjorie's negative automatic thoughts about herself, other people, and her future.

TREATMENT AIMS

We distinguish aims as small steps toward a larger overarching treatment goal. Bandura and Simon (1977) made a similar distinction between *end goals* (i.e., overarching goals) and *subgoals* (i.e., aims). Overarching end goals serve a general, directive function toward an aspiration (e.g., a more satisfying life), but they appear to have little impact on what individuals actually choose to do in the here and now. Subgoals (or aims) play a more central role in immediate behaviors and in how hard individuals will work on these behaviors (Bandura & Simon, 1977).

Even if end goals appear incredibly difficult to reach, people can maintain a high level of motivation through a progression of subgoals. Bandura and Simon (1977) argued that subgoals are most satisfying and motivating when they are somewhat challenging but still attainable. For many clients like Marjorie, it may be impossible to imagine that an end goal of "feeling better" will ever come to pass, because it is hard to imagine how to begin on the road to achieving that goal. However, gradually increasing pleasant activities seems more attainable, in part because of the greater specificity of these aims. In setting goals, the clinician's objective is to replace the overwhelming burden of wanting to feel better with a sense of working toward a manageable set of subgoals or aims.

The therapist works with the client to translate issues on the Problem List into realistic steps for treatment that represent the aims of each phase. Aims should be specific, concrete, and measurable. Hayes, Barlow, and Nelson-Gray (1999) suggest a variety of strategies to help clients refine the Problem List and move from abstract ideas to quantifiable objectives. These include asking clients to identify how they or someone else would know that their goal had been accomplished, or having them describe a *current* typical day versus an *ideal* typical day. Minimizing the discrepancy between these descriptions can serve as a treatment aim. Nelson (1981) recommends identifying either partial or instrumental goals rather than emphasizing a global objective. She describes an example in which the client's overall goal for treatment was to increase self-esteem, but the treatment initially focused on (and measured) the more instrumental aim of getting a raise at work.

Concrete aims are more likely than "vague intentions" to lead to actual behavior change (Bandura & Schunk, 1981). For example, Marjorie's therapist translated her overall goal of being less depressed into a number of aims, such as increasing her physical activity, regulating her sleep and eating schedules, improving her social support, and identifying and challenging her negative automatic thoughts. As we discuss in Chapter 4, another critical component of the PACC model is ongoing assessment, which requires measurable aims. Unless the aims are measurable, the client and therapist will have difficulty knowing when or if improvements are being made. Ideally, treatment aims should be relevant to the client's highest priority problem. Although the therapist and client can sometimes easily agree on which problem is the highest priority, at other times this can be challenging.

For example, Sid, a young adult newly diagnosed with bipolar disorder, began taking lithium approximately 2 months before entering psychotherapy. When asked to describe his goals for treatment, Sid replied, "To get off medication." The medication was a constant reminder of his illness, decreased his energy level, and made concentration difficult. His parents were also encouraging him to "stop putting chemicals" into his body. Sid was fairly responsive to the therapist's urging that he put off his decision about the medication until his body had time to adjust fully to the side effects and he had time to explore what it means to have bipolar disorder. The overarching goal of treatment shifted from "getting off medication" to "understanding bipolar illness."

In this case, the aims of the first phase of treatment included increased knowledge of medication and its side effects, psychoeducation about the etiology and prognosis of bipolar disorder, and the implementation of beneficial lifestyle changes, such as maintaining a regular sleep schedule. Sid pursued these aims using strategies such as reading psychoeducational materials, identifying and challenging negative appraisals about taking medications, exploring the impact that bipolar disorder was having on his hopes for the future, and exploring the impact that bipolar disorder was having on his relationships with others (e.g., family, friends, girlfriend).

Number of Aims

Although the number of aims is likely to vary per client, we generally suggest having about three aims in each phase of treatment. When a client and therapist have trouble generating more than one aim, the aim may not be specific enough. The therapist's challenge in such cases is to come up with concrete, specific aims when the client's treatment goal is vague (e.g., to feel "happier," "less anxious," or "more in control").

Having more than three aims, although not impossible, can be somewhat burdensome to the client and therapist, particularly if the aims cover numerous domains of functioning. For example, Sally, a 60-year-old woman, sought treatment for a depressive episode in the context of an impending separation from her partner. Her partner's primary reasons for wanting to separate were Sally's angry outbursts and verbal abuse. Sally reported a different perspective, seeing herself as weak, dependent, and unable to assert her own opinions. She also described herself as a failure, unable to hold down a steady job or maintain friendships. The therapist and Sally initially agreed upon four aims for the first phase of treatment shown in Figure 3.3.

When they began working on these aims, Sally and her therapist found themselves being pulled in multiple directions, ranging from discussions of the pros and cons of maintaining Sally's romantic relationship to her low self-esteem and inability to initiate new social contacts, to her increasing depressed mood and inability to get out of bed in the morning. After a few weeks, her therapist realized that it would be preferable to step back and work on one problem at a time. The therapist accordingly discussed with Sally the possibility of focusing just on her depressive symptoms at first, with the specific aims of regulating her sleep–wake cycle, pursuing pleasure and mastery activities, and identifying the beliefs that reinforced her negative self-view. Sally agreed not to make any major decisions about her future with her partner until some of her depressive symptoms had subsided. Over the next month, Sally was better able to focus her energies on alleviating

---

Treatment Phase I   **Date:** January 3, 2002

Aims: **1.** Learn new communication skills and implement them with partner.

2. Reduce daily anger outbursts.

3. Seek out new forms of social support, such as making new friends.

4. Increase involvement in activities that give pleasure and a sense of mastery.

Measures: **1.** _____
(attach graph)
2. _____

3. _____

Strategies: **1.** _____

2. _____

3. _____

Date for Phase I Progress Review: March 31, 2002

FIGURE 3.3. Aims of Phase I for Sally.

her depressed mood, and by the second phase of treatment, she began to work effectively on anger management and communication skills in the context of her relationship.

Disagreement about Aims

Some clients come to the first therapy session with aims for treatment that are different from those the therapist would advocate. Negotiating effective treatment plans with such clients can be difficult, sometimes resulting in the therapist walking a fine line between supporting versus contradicting the client's wishes. For example, Jane, a 20-year-old woman, presented with a 4-year history of bulimia nervosa, current major depression, and a recent suicide attempt. Jane's therapist was primarily concerned about her depressed mood, hopelessness, and ongoing suicidal thoughts. Jane, however, was interested only in the aim of maintaining or reducing her current body weight (which was average) and eliminating her binge-eating episodes.

In this case, the therapist believed that Jane's own treatment aims were secondary in importance to her depression and suicidal ideation. To foster a therapeutic alliance and productive working relationship with the client, the therapist was invested in developing a treatment aim that would be acceptable to Jane. In choosing to be open about the dilemma, she phrased it as follows:

> "I understand that the reason for your being in treatment right now is to maintain your current weight and to get rid of your nightly binges. I hear you saying how important these goals are, but I'm feeling worried because I am seriously concerned for your safety given your recent suicide attempt, and your feelings of sadness and hopelessness. I wonder if we could reach some sort of compromise in our aims for this phase of our treatment? In other words, could we agree to work at least initially on reducing your feelings of sadness and hopelessness and then turn to your binge eating and body image?

Jane agreed that this was a reasonable direction for the early phase of treatment. She contracted for safety with the therapist and agreed to make some behavioral changes (e.g., engaging in pleasant activities and keeping mood records) designed to change her depressed mood. She also made a commitment to begin eating three balanced meals a day as a step toward decreasing her urges to binge in the evenings. Although Jane never made a commitment *not* to focus on her weight, monitoring body weight was not included in the first phase of treatment. Over the course of this first phase, Jane's depressive symptoms decreased significantly. Her episodes of binge eating became somewhat less frequent, but her purging continued on an almost daily basis. Not until the second phase of treatment did Jane and her therapist begin working on the aims of improving her body image, eating a balanced diet, and reducing bingeing and purging overall.

Jane's case illustrates how the aggregate of aims over the course of multiple treatment phases can lead to achieving the larger treatment goal. In order to alleviate Jane's depressed mood as well as address her eating disorder, the therapist generated a variety of aims that were likely to cover multiple phases of treatment. The ultimate goals of Jane's therapy may have included eating more healthfully, being less critical of her body, and feeling happier, but progress toward such goals were made gradually, one step at a time.

TREATMENT STRATEGIES

When a practitioner takes the time to articulate the strategies to be used in pursuit of a given therapeutic aim, the strategies serve as guideposts to assist in staying focused. Explicitly planning strategies for each phase of treatment also facilitates the process of informed consent by helping clients to be aware of the approach the clinician is using and clarifying the rationale for its expected effectiveness. The more specific the treatment strategy, the better. Simply indicating "cognitive therapy" is not necessarily informative; entire books have been written on the different strategies this approach comprises. Instead, the therapist should attempt to articulate as concretely as possible what he or she will do to help the client make progress on the specified aims.

Selection of Treatment Strategies: The Use of Practice Guidelines

Once the clinician has established aims for a particular phase of treatment, how does he or she choose (or develop) a strategy to achieve them? One approach we favor, on both a convenience and scientific basis, is to apply a treatment guideline or tested treatment protocol. Although the research literature does not cover the rich complexity of all clinical issues, researchers have shown pretty conclusively that selected available treatments effectively ameliorate some specified disorders and problems. Furthermore, we can improve quality of care by using what we know from research about which interventions work better than others, and under what circumstances (O'Keefe, Quittner, & Melamed, 1996).

Professionals across the range of health care fields have begun to develop treatment guidelines in recognition of the need to use the research literature as a foundation of treatment planning. Hundreds of guidelines have been developed by professional organizations such as the American Psychiatric Association (e.g., American Psychiatric Association, 1993), by government initiatives such as the Australian Quality Assurance Project (e.g., Quality Assurance Project, 1982, 1985), and by provider organizations (e.g., managed care organizations, hospitals, and large group practices).

Other groups have provided lists of well-tested treatments for specific problems (e.g., Chambless et al., 1998). (This report is also available at *http://pantheon.yale.edu/~tat22//est_docs/ValidatedTx.pdf*. A user-friendly version with links to informative websites is located at *http://www.apa.org/divisions/div12/rev_est/index.shtml*.) The Cochrane Collaboration has steadily expanded its user-friendly database on reviews of treatment literature to include topics in mental health (it does not actually prepare practice guidelines but systematically reviews the empirical literature to guide practitioners in their choices). The Cochrane Library is accessible from most university libraries at *www.update-software.com/cochrane*. An analogous and helpful database that has been developed by the Campbell Collaboration (see *http://campbell.gse.upenn.edu/*) includes a set of systematic reviews of studies on the effects of social and educational policies and practices.

We strongly encourage the use of empirically supported treatments where they are available. The treatments are often a basis for practice guidelines, which ideally rely on the research literature and also take into account the setting and practical constraints. For example, the treatment with the best research support for a given problem may also require expertise that is unavailable in a particular setting, or the cost of a particular treatment may place it out of reach in some settings. Practice guidelines are good resources for busy practitioners, because they do not require synthesizing the research literature in order to have a scientific basis for practice (Kirk, 1999). We have found practice guidelines particularly helpful for the PACC approach, because they offer clear recommendations about which treatment strategies to use.

Shifting Strategies over the Course of Treatment

Therapy is liable to take a number of unexpected twists and turns, often prompted by a client's life events, such as job loss, death of a loved one, or breakup of a romantic relationship. If the change is particularly dramatic, the therapist and client may decide to begin a new phase of treatment, complete with a new set of aims and strategies. However, if the change is compatible with the current treatment aims, then it is often beneficial to continue with the same set of aims but slightly revised treatment strategies.

Consider the following case example illustrating revision of strategies during a therapy phase. Beth, a 30-year-old woman, entered therapy to address feelings of worthlessness and uncertainty about her future with her boyfriend. Her primary aim during the first phase of treatment was related to her romantic relationship. Specifically, she placed a high priority on being "less of a pushover" with her boyfriend and feeling "more confident" as a romantic partner. One of the initial treatment strategies was to help Beth identify her own desires and needs in the relationship and to practice talking about these needs with her boyfriend. When she and her boyfriend broke up, Beth and her therapist felt that she should continue to practice skills related to assertiveness with other people in her life. The earlier treatment strategies were modified to be compatible with Beth's current situation.

Specifically, the therapist began to teach more general communication skills (e.g., active listening, use of "I" statements), so that Beth could work on assertiveness in the context of other relationships (e.g., coworkers and friends instead of her boyfriend). In some cases, a few sessions may be needed to build the bridge between the current crisis and the Treatment Plan. Beth spent two sessions exploring emotions related to her breakup, affirming that the decision to break up was a healthy one that enhanced rather than impeded her treatment goals. The transition back to the original Treatment Plan was relatively smooth, and Beth was actively involved in the treatment-related decision-making process.

Flexibility of Treatment Strategies

Sometimes therapists need flexibility in the type of strategy used to accomplish the treatment aim. For example, a patient with panic disorder may have a paradoxical reaction to progressive muscle relaxation; that is, although relaxation training is intended to reduce anxiety overall, some clients actually become more, rather than less, anxious during this exercise. In response, the therapist may attempt another treatment strategy, such as diaphragmatic breathing, in order to reduce anxiety. If the client has a paradoxical reaction to diaphragmatic breathing as well (as do some of our clients), the treatment strategy may then need to be changed to guided imagery of relaxing scenes. In subtle variations in the type of strategy to accomplish the aim of the current phase of treatment (e.g., relaxation training), it is not necessary to change phases of treatment or to make major changes in the Treatment Plan. Instead, new strategies can be added to the current phase of treatment.

The strategies can branch across theoretical orientations. The PACC approach encourages flexibility in the types of aims and strategies used in treatment, and it is our belief that one's theoretical orientation need not prohibit use of these treatment-planning techniques. The goal is to use an evidence-based approach to select the first line of treatment strategies, rather than feeling restricted by a particular theoretical orientation. Naturally, case conceptualizations from some orientations will more readily translate into specific measurable aims, but for the reasons discussed earlier, we believe the effort to specify aims and strategies is worthwhile in all cases.

CHOOSING AIMS AND STRATEGIES: CASE EXAMPLE

Jean, a hairdresser, presented to the clinic reporting trouble controlling her spending. Despite being able to control spending for food and clothing for her family, she had spent $4,000 over the past year on paraphernalia associated with basketball and stuffed animals for her home. She also mentioned that her shopping was having a negative impact on her marriage. Based on Jean's initial evaluation, a Treatment Plan was developed to reduce her impulsive spending through cognitive and behavioral interventions. Specifically, the first aim was to reduce the number of impulse purchases Jean made per week, with the expected goal of cutting her purchases by 50% from baseline within 6 weeks (see Figure 3.2). A review date was scheduled for this 6-week time point, and weekly progress on this aim was graphed for easy visual reference. The strategies to meet this aim included developing cognitive counters to her automatic thoughts about the imperative of buying things sold at a good price, as well as initiating behavioral interventions to limit cues and opportunities for buying. For example, Jean agreed not to carry a credit card, to restrict her time in stores, and to make lists of acceptable purchases as a way to help set limits.

Both Jean and her therapist agreed to this treatment plan. However, just a few weeks into treatment, it became apparent that her marriage was in serious trouble, and the spending was only one of the problems impacting her relationship. Jean was able to bring her shopping under control faster than anticipated, but she was having great difficulty with her spouse. Although the review date had not yet arrived, the therapist reformulated the Treatment Plan to reflect the new information and Jean's changing priorities with respect to the difficulties with her marriage. The plan for the second phase focused on fostering assertive communication patterns with her husband (while continuing to monitor spending behaviors for signs of a lapse), and the therapist established a new review date.

Jean's rapid transition to a new treatment phase illustrates the need to shift the treatment focus when a problem ranked low in priority becomes more pressing than the one previously targeted. In addition, this shift emphasizes the need to choose aims relevant to the highest priority problem presented by the client. Furthermore, this case illustrates the need to return to the Problem List, set new aims, plan new measurement approaches, and implement new therapeutic strategies when the focus of treatment changes. Figure 3.4 shows the full Treatment Plan for Jean in these two phases.

CHALLENGES IN IMPLEMENTING THE TREATMENT PLAN

Pursuing a Collaborative Endeavor

Collaboration with clients, a central feature of many models of psychotherapy, is certainly compatible with the PACC approach to treatment planning. Although collaboration involves challenges, the benefits are numerous. Some evidence indicates that operating in a more collaborative style leads to measurably better treatment outcomes (Whiston & Sexton, 1993) and that clients benefit from open discussion of their role in therapy (Eisenberg, 1981; Friedlander, 1981). Furthermore, clients who are treated as partners in the therapeutic endeavor are more likely to experience a sense of agency in the pursuit of their goals. Using data from his own protocol for treatment planning, Bernstein (1992) writes, "I have been particularly impressed with the many innovative ideas the clients have contributed to their own treatment designs. Rather than feeling restricted (as I had feared) by the concreteness of their treatment plans, their awareness of the process stimulated their curiosity and problem-solving abilities" (p. 272).

Treatment Phase I	Date: January 20, 2002

Aims: **1.** Reduce the frequency of impulse purchases per week.

2. Reduce believability of maladaptive ideas like, "I must take advantage of sale prices."

3. Reduce time spent ruminating about money.

Measures:
(attach graph)

1. Amount of money spent on impulse purchases per week

2. Y-BOCS Compulsive spending checklist

3. Self-reported distress (on a 0–100 scale) and time spent thinking about money

Strategies: **1.** Develop cognitive counters to Jean's automatic thoughts about buying.

2. Limit buying cues & opportunities (e.g., no credit cards, restrict time in stores).

3. Make lists of acceptable purchases to help Jean set limits.

Date for Phase I Progress Review: March 2, 2002

Treatment Phase II	Date: February 10, 2002

Aims: **1.** Reduce anxiety level and rumination about marital relationship throughout the day.

2. Communicate more assertively with husband.

3. Maintain gains made in reducing spending behavior.

Measures:
(attach graph)

1. Daily average anxiety level and time spent ruminating about the relationship

2. Positive–negative weekly checklist of assertive responding

3. Amount of money spent on impulse purchases per week

Strategies: **1.** Identify and challenge negative automatic thoughts about marital relationship.

2. Use assertiveness training to meet her needs without escalating conflict.

3. Teach progressive muscle relaxation in order to reduce overall anxiety level.

Date for Phase II Progress Review: April 20, 2002

FIGURE 3.4. Phase I and II Treatment Plan for Jean.

A collaborative approach to treatment planning can also empower the client. Clients who adopt a problem-solving attitude toward treatment become more actively engaged in therapy and experience a better outcome (Luborsky, Crits-Cristoph, Mintz, & Auerbach, 1988). Most individuals enter therapy when they find themselves confused about their problems or unable to take action to address them. Through an open negotiation of treatment goals, the therapist can foster the client's potential to deal with problems more effectively (McConnaughy, DiClemente, Prochaska, & Velicer, 1989). Therapeutic outcome improves when clients perceive they have a choice in the therapeutic process and are knowledgeable about therapy options (Brehm & Smith, 1986). Furthermore, clients are more likely to adhere to treatment and maintain health-related behaviors when they feel a personal commitment to the Treatment Plan (Putnam, Finney, Barkley, & Bonner, 1994).

Of course, sharing the treatment-planning process with clients and maintaining their commitment to the treatment goals can be difficult depending on the characteristics of the client. Persons (1989) recommends that therapists refrain from discussing the Treatment Plan in great detail with people with obsessive personalities, because these clients are likely to retard progress by focusing too much on minute details of the plan. With obsessive clients, it may be best to present the Treatment Plan one therapy phase at a time (Bernstein, 1992).

Collaborative treatment planning can also be challenging with clients who begin therapy with unrealistically high expectations for change and a rigid desire to tackle multiple domains at once. One strategy for facing such challenges is to incorporate the client's difficulties with unrealistic expectations and rigidity into the Treatment Plan. For example, Lea, a client who began a new phase of psychotherapy with high expectations for change and perfectionistic standards, was a 40-year-old, single woman with a history of four inpatient hospitalizations for bipolar disorder. After Lea's most recent hospitalization, she attended a day treatment program emphasizing psychoeducation and cognitive and behavioral problem-solving skills. This form of treatment was new to Lea, but it appealed to her.

After completing the day treatment program, Lea began working with a new individual therapist. When asked to describe her goals for treatment, Lea produced a list of 30 items, including "eliminating my drive for perfectionism," "learning to see the glass as half full rather than as half empty," and "increasing self-confidence in interpersonal interactions." Lea had great difficulty prioritizing the goals on her list.

She said, "Each item is just as important as the next. I can't imagine picking one goal over the other, because I'm not sure which will help me the most, and I have to prevent myself from going downhill again." Continued discussion over the next two sessions allowed Lea to identify how her perfectionistic standards were preventing her from narrowing down her expectations. Setting a limited number of reasonable goals for herself at the beginning of each week became one of Lea's aims in the first phase of treatment.

Challenges in sharing the treatment-planning process can also arise with clients who have difficulty identifying overarching treatment goals or for whom all problems appear to have an external explanation. For example, Neal, a 25-year-old male with an atypical anxiety disorder and a narcissistic personality style, came to treatment with the goal of "managing anxiety." Collaborative treatment planning became challenging, however, when Neal described his anxiety as being due mostly to his concern with "other people's issues." Specifically, Neal described himself as "independent" and "insightful" and other people as "passive" and "troubled." At the start of treatment, Neal was uninterested in examining his interactions with others or his thoughts about the roles he played in other people's lives. Instead, he was committed to the idea that if he could get the people around him to change how they behaved, then his own anxiety would subside. Neal and his therapist were able to agree that one step toward relieving his anxiety was to identify when and under what circumstances his anxiety was at its worst. Two of Neal's treatment aims were to recognize interpersonal triggers of anxiety and to reduce time spent ruminating about interpersonal relationships.

Many clients do hold unrealistic goals for treatment. Whereas Lea's unrealistic goal setting appeared to come from her perfectionistic standards, Neal's unrealistic goals came from his lack of insight into his own role in his relations with other people. Another difficulty that sometimes arises in collaboratively setting goals occurs when clients are not yet prepared or committed to make changes. In this case, the therapist's initial aim is for the client to become motivated and ready to change, but the client may not yet be aware of his or her ambivalence toward change.

Motivation and Readiness for Change

Not all clients are intrinsically motivated to make changes in their lives. Sometimes the reasons for resistance to change are clear, such as when an individual is court-referred or sent to treatment by a parent or guardian. Resistance is especially common in addiction problems, domestic violence, and problems in which at least some of the symptoms are considered to be positive by the client (such as low body weight in anorexia).

An important consideration in collaborative treatment is the client's readiness for change (DiClemente, 1991; DiClemente, Prochaska, & Gilbertini, 1985; Prochaska, DiClemente, & Norcross, 1992). As DiClemente (1991) describes, "A therapist can be understood as a midwife to the process of change, which has its own unique course in each case. Skillful therapists will best facilitate change if they understand the process of change and learn how to activate or instigate the unfolding of that process" (p. 191). In part, the therapist's job is to recognize a client's ambivalence and tailor the intervention to the client's stage of change.

Various modifications of the stages of change model have occurred since its initial development by Prochaska and DiClemente (1982); research has supported the predictive utility of the more recent version (Prochaska & DiClemente, 1992). In the *precontemplation* stage, the individual has no plan to change behavior in the near future (typically, the next 6 months) and may lack awareness about the severity of his or her problem. Direct attempts to change behavior at this stage will frequently be met with resistance. During *contemplation*, the individual acknowledges the existence of the problem and is seriously thinking about taking steps to work on it, but he or she has not yet made a commitment to take action. At this point, it is common for the client to struggle with a cost–benefit analysis of maintaining versus finding a solution to the problem.

In the *preparation* stage, the person not only intends to change (typically, within the next month) but also has made some actual attempt to change the behavior during the previous year. Usually, individuals in this stage have already made a small reduction in the problem behavior (e.g., smoking five fewer cigarettes per day) but are not quite ready to take effective action. In contrast, during the *action* stage, individuals modify their behavior, experiences, or environment to overcome their problems. This process usually requires overt efforts to change that involve substantial time and energy. Finally, in the *maintenance* stage, the individual works to stabilize the changes made during the action stage and to prevent relapses from occurring. This stage signifies a continuation of change rather than a static phase or final event. It is not unusual for clients to repeat these five stages in a spiral pattern before the maintenance phase is sustained.

Stage models of change may be useful as a heuristic to help guide treatment planning. Prochaska (1991) urges clinicians to match the therapeutic intervention to the client's stage of change. For example, Prochaska suggests that if a client is in a precontemplation stage, then the wisest course may be therapeutic intervention that focuses primarily on consciousness raising. In contrast, if this person is in an action stage, behavioral procedures are likely to capitalize on client readiness. In the context of treatment planning, the types of aims and strategies that the client is likely to find appealing will shift over time, perhaps as readiness for change shifts over time. Clients experiencing symptoms for the first time (e.g., a client who is experiencing his first manic episode) or those in treatment only to appease others or to satisfy a mandate (e.g., from the court) are least likely to be ready to change. The effectiveness of treatment may depend upon first enhancing the client's commitment to therapy.

Miller and Rollnick (1991) argue that it is detrimental to the treatment-planning process to conceptualize a lack of motivation as "denial," "resistance," or "a personality problem." Instead, they describe motivation as a state that fluctuates across time and situations. Motivation, when thought of as a state rather than a trait, can be influenced. Miller and Rollnick argue that assessing and influencing motivation is "an inherent and central part of the professional's task" (p. 19). These authors have developed a protocol for motivational interviewing that we have found very helpful in getting clients "unstuck" from their ambivalence, so that they can make positive changes.

Axis II Factors and Conditions

Some clients have long-standing interpersonal styles or personality traits that result in resistance to changing an Axis I problem. For others, the style or trait may itself be the problem that is the focus of treatment. Personality disorders are relatively common, with prevalence estimated at 10–18% for the general population (see Turner & Dudek, 1997), and perhaps higher among outpatients at mental health clinics. Practitioners have long observed the complexity and challenge presented by patients with personality disorders. Because Axis II problems are by definition central to the person's identity (representing pervasive and enduring ways of thinking and behaving), changes occur more slowly than changes in Axis I problems. This reality has a direct impact on treatment planning. Assessments of clients being treated for Axis II disorders are likely to be spaced farther apart, and changes may be more subtle and cumulative.

Although measurement of Axis II conditions has proven more difficult and unwieldy than assessment of Axis I symptoms, reputable indices and even core testing batteries do exist. For example, Strupp, Horowitz, and Lambert (1997) include reviews and recommendations regarding several useful assessment tools. We encourage clinicians to consider measuring Axis II conditions even if they are not the explicit focus of clinical interventions. By monitoring Axis II conditions, clinicians will have a clearer idea of the possible explanations when a treatment for Axis I problems proves ineffectual.

SHORTCUTS FOR THE BUSY CLINICIAN

Generating treatment aims and strategies may be more straightforward in some cases than others. Many clinicians juggle large caseloads, and developing a written Treatment Plan may initially seem to be an unmanageable burden. To assist with this process, we have generated an initial (though certainly not comprehensive) list of treatment aims and strategies for the busy clinician, based on the biopsychosocial Problem List described in Chapter 2 (see Table 3.1). Earlier in this chapter, we included information for accessing several websites that provide information on empirically supported treatments. Information about access to treatment manuals for some of these treatments is available at *http://pantheon.yale.edu/~tat22//est_docs/ValidatedTx.pdf*. Finally, we recommend consulting *A Guide to Treatments That Work*, edited by Nathan and Gorman (2002), for additional direction in selecting empirically supported aims and strategies, and also *Treatments of Psychiatric Disorders*, edited by Gabbard (2001), developed by the American Psychiatric Association.

TABLE 3.1. Examples of Treatment Aims and Strategies across Domains of Functioning

Problem domain	Treatment aims	Treatment strategies
Clinical Crises	Reduce frequency and intensity of suicidal thoughts.	Develop a crisis plan including warning signs, coping strategies, and emergency supports.
	Reduce frequency and intensity of homicidal thoughts.	Develop a crisis plan including triggers, coping strategies, and emergency supports.
	Reduce frequency of self-injurious behavior.	Create an impulse control plan.
School/ occupational functioning and finances	Make short-term career choices and take steps to pursue career goals.	Consider pros and cons of potential career choices.
	Increase weekly attendance at job/school.	Develop a weekly schedule including rewards for meeting obligations.
	Decrease spending sprees and increase financial independence.	Create a budget and develop strategies to diminish buying urges.
Family functioning	Reduce frequency of arguments with family members.	Improve understanding of interpersonal dynamics fueling conflicts.
	Improve marital communication.	Learn to express needs and desires assertively.
	Understand (and limit) impact of trauma history on current family functioning.	Learn safety cues and discuss impact of trauma on current view of self.
	Increase parenting self-efficacy and reduce the use of corporal punishment.	Learn parenting management skills.
Extrafamily interpersonal functioning	Enhance sense of self as an independent and competent individual.	Practice making autonomous decisions daily.
	Decrease social isolation.	Phone one friend each week.
	Decrease social anxiety.	Practice relaxation techniques and gradual exposure daily.
	Improve social network by exploring community resources.	Visit one new community organization weekly.
	Cope with interpersonal stressors of separation and loss.	Explore spiritual and existential avenues of making meaning out of loss.

(continued)

Problem domain	Treatment aims	Treatment strategies
Behavioral health	Increase physical fitness and exercise frequency.	Join an athletic club; develop an exercise routine and exercise three times a week.
	Improve nutrition and food choices.	Receive psychoeducation about nutrition.
	Maintain a regular eating schedule.	Plan daily menus and use food records.
	Reduce frequency of binge or purge episodes.	Implement regular eating, decision delay strategies; understand interpersonal dynamics fueling eating disorder.
	Improve health-seeking behavior (e.g., medical treatment compliance, psychiatric consultation).	Make appointments to meet with health care professionals.
	Increase compliance with medication.	Create a behavioral schedule that includes medication.
	Improve stress management skills.	Learn relaxation techniques and practice daily.
	Reduce frequency of legal drug use (e.g., caffeine, nicotine, prescription drugs, diet medications).	Create behavioral targets; attend relevant support groups (e.g., smoking cessation).
Risky behaviors	Decrease alcohol use by 50%.	Examine triggers for drinking; attend support group meetings (e.g., AA) weekly.
	Abstain from drugs.	Monitor urges and cravings; identify triggers and warning signs; practice relapse prevention skills.
	Decrease frequency of risky sexual behaviors.	Receive psychoeducation about safer sexual behaviors.
	Decrease frequency of gambling episodes.	Set a spending limit for gambling each week.
	Decrease risky or thrill-seeking behaviors.	Develop an impulse control plan and practice skills daily.
Cultural, spiritual, and moral development	Increase acceptance of the role of cultural challenges in current functioning.	Speak with close family members about their own struggles with cultural identity (e.g., biculturalism, acculturation, ethnic identity).
	Develop a renewed sense of self as a spiritual individual.	Increase–decrease involvement with religious institutions.
	Enhance understanding of existential issues.	Keep a journal describing existential questions and challenges.
	Gain confidence in coping with moral dilemmas and issues.	Learn decision-making skills and apply them to moral dilemmas and issues.

CHAPTER 4

ONGOING
MEASUREMENT

Some clinicians are reluctant even to consider the idea of measurement. As Gottman and Leiblum (1974) quipped, "We realize that many therapists are about as interested in the evaluation of psychotherapy as they are in having someone else judge the quality of their lovemaking" (p. 2). Measuring progress throughout treatment may at first seem daunting and even sterile, removed in some way from the valuable relationship between the therapist and the client. However, many of the common concerns about measuring progress (e.g., that it entails a large time commitment or great knowledge of statistics) are simply myths. Relying on data to plan treatment does not mean that numbers are more important than clients. In contrast, structured measurement opens new possibilities for clients to express their experience of treatment.

Although most therapists have a sense of how their clients are doing, intuition is not the optimal guide for effective treatment planning. Evaluating progress without using actual measures is likely to be unreliable, and this problem undoubtedly grows along with the size of the clinician's caseload. Furthermore, most clients have problems that impact on several domains of their functioning. With many clients to attend to, and many problems for each client, it is no wonder that clinicians tend to rely on heuristics, or cognitive "rules of thumb," for estimating client status or change (Dawes, 1994; Meehl, 1973). Without being aware of it, everyone relies on these mental shortcuts to make all kinds of decisions. Most commonly, judgments are based on recall of instances similar to the current situation, or on expectations rather than on all of the available information. As important as clinical judgment is, research has shown that trained therapists do not have superior clinical predictive abilities compared to untrained persons (Goldberg, 1959). Fortunately, therapists *can* boost the reliability and validity of assessment by relying on established measures and actuarial methods when they are available (see Dawes, 1994; Wiggins, 1973).

Throughout this chapter, we provide information on measures that we have found to be useful in various settings in which we have worked. In selecting measures to discuss, we have been guided by the recommendations of Andrews, Peters, and Teesson (1994). Accordingly, we discuss measures with useful qualities in most clinical settings. We chose measures that are *applicable*, in the sense that they address variables that are both important to the client (such as symptoms, functioning, and satisfaction with services), and important to the clinician in formulating and implementing a Treatment Plan. We also aimed for measures that are *acceptable*, meaning brief and user-friendly, and *practical*. Practical measures involve minimal cost and have relatively simple scoring and interpretation; measures that require specialized training for use and interpretation are less practical. Finally, we tried to ensure that the measures we recommend evidence *reliability*, *validity*, and *sensitivity to treatment change*.

BENEFITS OF ONGOING MEASUREMENT

Most clinicians conduct initial assessments to evaluate the nature and severity of a client's problems. Clinicians who work in settings with some type of outcomes management, program evaluation, or research project may also do a brief assessment at the end of treatment. The value of the initial evaluation is clear to most clinicians, because it provides information necessary for treatment planning. The final assessment is useful for evaluating the relative success of the treatment, but it obviously does not directly facilitate treatment planning, because the treatment is finished at the time of the final evaluation. Conducting assessment as an ongoing process throughout treatment provides continuous feedback about the course of treatment progress and how well the changes generalize to other areas of client functioning. We briefly describe some of the key advantages of ongoing measurement, including the ways evaluation can improve treatment and enhance accountability. For a fuller discussion of these issues, see Hayes et al., (1999).

Ongoing measurement is useful whether the results are positive or negative. Perhaps most importantly, continuous measurement of progress allows the therapist to detect when an intervention fails to promote hoped-for changes. The therapist can then use this information to change strategies promptly. Directly measuring the acute problem(s) can also reassure the clinician when the specific goals of treatment are being met. Because clients often enjoy the process of therapy and want to reinforce the therapist's efforts, some may express satisfaction with a treatment even if it is ineffective for the targeted clinical problem. In contrast, other clients who fail to notice incremental gains expect to feel "normal" immediately, and so may continue to feel demoralized even when they are actually getting better. Both symptom change and global functioning are critical outcome measures, and sharing the results of ongoing assessment with clients can facilitate many types of therapy.

Measuring progress is consistent with a consumer-oriented approach, which values clients' views of their experiences and symptoms (Morrison, 1984). When measurement is incorporated into therapy, clients have a clear voice and a collaborative role in their own change process. Some evidence indicates that therapy outcome is improved when therapists give clients explicit feedback about their progress (Miller & Sovereign, 1989). Ongoing assessment may also help forestall burnout, because both the clinician and client can see regular, concrete markers of progress (Morrison, 1984). Regular measurement reassures clinicians that although therapy is often a bumpy road, changes do occur. Even when assessment shows no change or decreased functioning, the practice of regular measurement provides ongoing motivation for the therapist to engage problem-solving strategies and to reconsider the case conceptualization or Treatment Plan in response to the lack of progress.

In addition to the client's focal problems, the clinician can measure other important characteristics of the intervention, for example, evaluating the degree of client compliance with between-session recommendations. The most common area of compliance that we tend to monitor is the amount of medication a client takes, even those taken on an "as needed" basis. Compliance is also pertinent with regard to the practice of new skills, ranging from stress management (e.g., setting limits with regard to overtime at work) to basic skills of daily living (e.g., learning to use money and make change). To the extent that the therapist believes a given strategy will inspire positive change, it is important to assess the degree to which the client is actually using the strategy.

Assessing progress is not always straightforward, and it does require some investment of time at the outset. Once a measurement system is established, however, significant benefits accrue from knowing with confidence how much progress a client is making. Table 4.1 reviews some of the costs and benefits of conducting ongoing measurement of progress.

Measurement of progress does not remove the creative, personal aspects of psychotherapy. In fact, measuring abstract goals simply provides a greater challenge to creativity as therapists are pressured to define their constructs clearly. Consider for example spiritual development, which is often an important goal in transcendental/humanistic therapies. One of our clients who entered treatment was distressed about his growing ambivalence concerning involvement in his church and expressed a desire to expand his sense of spirituality in new directions. His therapist assessed spirituality using the short form of the Daily Spiritual Experiences scale (DSE; Underwood, 1999) and a weekly record of new spiritual activities. (The DSE, discussed in greater detail in Chapter 7, is included in the Appendix.) By interweaving creativity, client goals, and measurement in clinical practice, we provide better service to clients and promote public understanding of the value of our work.

TABLE 4.1. Benefits and Costs of Measuring Progress

Benefits

Enhances ability to track progress for multiple clients
Guides treatment planning based on data
Represents a client-centered approach to practice
Reduces the need to rely on memory
Encourages a rapid response to unproductive strategies
Facilitates change by providing feedback
Enhances accountability
Demonstrates effectiveness of treatment to relevant third parties
Documents assessment results
Motivates the therapist and clients
Other: _____

Costs

Time investment (especially up front)
Cost (depends on the measure)
Compliance can be a challenge for some clients
Difficulty obtaining some measures
Other: _____

OBSTACLES TO ROUTINE MEASUREMENT

Probably the biggest obstacle to conducting ongoing assessment is the perception that it will be time-consuming and costly. However, many assessment tools are available at no cost, requiring little time to administer and interpret. Throughout this chapter, we provide examples of tools that we have found helpful in practice. Later in the chapter, we also provide a list of websites, databases, and reference books that provide access to other measures. Once a library of low-cost instruments is established, there is minimal recurring time or expense. Some measures are worthwhile even if they are less convenient or more costly, because they provide such valuable information for treatment planning; these measures are typically administered less frequently.

Certainly, one obstacle that does occasionally arise is client resistance. In our experience, most clients respond positively to the concept of keeping records about different aspects of their problems. Some clients, however, are noncompliant with the therapist's request to complete questionnaires or self-monitoring forms. Obviously, clients are more likely to complete assessments that are straightforward and manageable. We strive to limit client assessment activities to just a few minutes a day, although some between-session exercises (i.e., intervention rather than assessment) may take longer. To illustrate, let us introduce the case of Thomas.

Thomas, a 35-year-old, single man, worked nights unloading and stocking merchandise at a large home improvement store. He sought treatment for depression exacerbated by his increasing social isolation and difficulty managing his anger. Thomas described himself as a very shy person and reported that he always had difficulty sticking up for himself. He thought his coworkers took him for granted and believed he was a much more conscientious and dedicated worker than the other men who worked the night shift. Thomas never talked with anyone about the frustration he felt at work. Immediately prior to seeking treatment, he found himself picking fights with his coworkers (both verbal and physical) with little provocation. Thomas believed that his anger was "completely out of control," and that he was destined to "erupt, totally out of the blue" for the rest of his life.

Part of the therapist's measurement plan was to monitor the frequency of anger outbursts Thomas experienced each day. Thomas was initially hesitant to keep track of his anger, in part because he was concerned that his depression would get worse as a result of having to count the number of times he "lost it" each day. The therapist explained that Thomas would not only be counting the number of anger outbursts but also working to better understand his feelings and control his behavior. The therapist gave Thomas an Anger Diary, which he agreed to complete daily. Figure 4.1 shows the Anger Diary, along with one of Thomas's entries.

Generally speaking, clients are more likely to be compliant if they buy into the rationale and utility of the assessment. In addition to simply explaining these ideas, the therapist can make them more vivid by reviewing and using assessment results within the session. For example, Thomas's therapist devised his Anger Diary primarily because she was interested in keeping track of the frequency and intensity of his anger episodes. Nevertheless, she also included assessment of other facets of anger that would provide information she felt would be useful during the sessions, such as triggers for anger, anger-related behaviors and cognitions, and how other people responded to Thomas's expression of anger.

Trigger	Anger Intensity (1–100)	Thoughts	Behavior	Consequences	Alternative Behavior
Coworker spills coffee on break and doesn't clean up.	85	He expects me to clean up his mess. Everyone always takes me for granted.	Swear at coworker and shove him as I walk by.	He and the other guys call me crazy and then leave me alone.	Ask coworker to please take care of his mess.

FIGURE 4.1. Thomas's Anger Diary.

Sometimes self-monitoring is a big task. Perhaps the most daunting example is a food diary. Just try keeping a record of everything you eat or drink for a week! (See Figure 4.2 for an example.) Food diaries commonly used to assess eating patterns among clients with eating disorders provide valuable information to the client and therapist, but they are onerous. For clients who feel overwhelmed by self-monitoring, we have found it helpful to break a large self-monitoring task (such as recording every morsel they eat) into smaller segments to help it seem less daunting. One strategy in this case is to ask the client to complete records for only 2 days the first week rather than every day. This information is then reviewed during the next session, so that the client can see how the information will be useful in the treatment. If the first week is successful, the client can keep the diary for 3 or 4 days the next week. For a client who continues to be noncompliant, alternative forms of assessment have to be considered, or a partner or teacher can be enlisted (with appropriate consent) to assist the client with the monitoring.

Without a doubt, some measures developed and used in research are impractical, because they are expensive, time-consuming to administer and interpret, or because they are published in outlets generally unavailable to practitioners. For example, psychophysiological measures often require specialized equipment or expertise. Throughout this chapter, we include measures that are in the public domain (i.e., free to use). Practitioners in solo practice often form cooperative peer groups to share assessment tools that must be purchased. (Some of these sources are listed in the Appendix.) Most of the strategies we recommend, however, do not involve extensive assessment kits. When it seems that there is no existing measure to meet the measurement need, clinicians can also design a tool tailored to the particular client, although this is less ideal because of the obvious concerns about reliability and validity.

COMPLETING THE MEASURES SECTION
OF THE TREATMENT PHASE FORM

The measures section of the treatment phase form is most helpful for treatment planning if specific measures are detailed in advance. Writing something like "evaluate depression" or "assess anger control" is not as helpful as "complete the Beck Depression Inventory weekly" or "maintain a daily frequency count of anger outbursts in the classroom

Day	Time	Food/Beverages & Portion Size
Monday 6/8/01	9:15 A.M. 1:00 P.M. 3:00 P.M. 6:45 P.M.	2 slices toast w. peanut butter, 1 cup pineapple, 10 oz. black tea, 8 oz. OJ 1 c. rice, 1 c. curried veggies, can of Nestea caramel rice cake, herbal tea 2 c. pasta w. tofu, 1 c. salad w. lemon & olive oil dressing, 5 oz. red wine
Tuesday		
Wednesday		
Thursday		
Friday		
Saturday		
Sunday		

FIGURE 4.2. Daily Food Record.

91

and at home, based on parent and teacher observations." In our own practice, we aim for about three measures for each client, with the assumption that some of the measures will be administered more frequently and others less so. In order to illustrate the way measurement is included in treatment planning, we provide a case example.

Doug, a 52-year-old, married, unemployed man originally from the Middle East, had a lifelong history of drug and alcohol abuse, and a current major depressive episode. The first phase of Doug's treatment focused almost exclusively on his major depressive episode and lack of activity (see Figure 4.3 for Doug's Treatment Plan). Measurements in the first phase of treatment included the Center for Epidemiologic Studies Depression scale (CES-D; Radloff, 1977; see Appendix), chosen by Doug's therapist because it is a reliable and valid measure of depressive symptoms with cross-cultural norms, and free and available to the public. Doug also monitored the number of pleasant activities he carried out each day and the quality of his sleep (see Figure 4.4). After 3 months of treatment, Doug was experiencing far fewer depressive symptoms and had acquired a part-time job in retail. However, he reported increasing tensions with his wife, prompted in part by his alcohol consumption and perceived inability to communicate effectively with her.

Although Doug denied suicidal ideation, his therapist might have chosen to include the Hopelessness Scale (Beck, Weissman, Lester, & Trexler, 1974), along with the daily activity log and sleep diary, had these facets of depression been important for Doug. The Hopelessness Scale, which takes about 5 minutes for the client to complete, has been shown to be predictive of subsequent suicide attempts and correlates with suicidal ideation and intent. Information about obtaining the Beck Hopelessness Scale (and the popular Beck Depression Inventory) is included in the Appendix. With a multimeasure approach, the assessment tools can precisely reflect the client's problems.

In the second phase of treatment, Doug's therapist continued to monitor his depressive symptoms using the CES-D, but because the aims of treatment had changed, the measures changed as well. Doug began monitoring his daily alcohol intake and marital satisfaction. The therapist asked Doug to use a self-recording card (McCrady, 1993) to monitor his urges to drink and the type and number of alcoholic beverages he actually consumed (see Figure 4.5). On a weekly basis, Doug also completed the Kansas Marital Satisfaction scale (KMS; Schumm et al., 1986; see Appendix), a 3-item scale in the public domain that correlates highly ($r = .83$) with the well-known Dyadic Adjustment Scale

Treatment Phase I   **Date:** March 31, 2002

Aims: **1.** Reduce depressive symptoms by 50%.

   2. Engage in at least 2 pleasurable activities every day.

   3. Normalize sleep schedule: regular bedtime and waking time, at least 7 hours of sleep each night, only one nap (planned in advance) each day.

Measures: **1.** Center for Epidemiologic Studies Depression scale (weekly)
(attach graph)
   2. Number of pleasant activities (daily)

   3. Number of hours and quality of sleep (daily)

Strategies: **1.** Daily behavioral scheduling (including time with wife, exercise, phone calls to friends, reading, job searching)

   2. Monitor and challenge negative automatic thoughts (e.g., I'm a failure; I can't do anything right; I don't deserve anything in life)

   3. Relaxation skills (deep breathing, meditation)

Date for Phase I Progress Review: June 30, 2002

Treatment Phase II   **Date:** July 1, 2002

Aims: **1.** Reduce depressive symptoms by an additional 10%.

   2. Reduce alcohol consumption by 25%.

   3. Engage in at least two pleasurable activities with wife each week.

Measures: **1.** Center for Epidemiologic Studies Depression scale (every 2 weeks)
(attach graph)
   2. Self-recording card of urges and drinks (daily)

   3. Kansas Marital Satisfaction Scale (weekly)

Strategies: **1.** Impulse control planning (when urge to drink occurs engage in distraction activities, journaling, leave the house, go to AA or NA, etc.)

   2. Communication skills training (e.g., increase "I" statements, ability to be assertive, willingness to compromise)

   3. Monitor and challenge negative automatic thoughts related to marriage (e.g., I can never live up to my wife's expectations; I'm unlovable)

Date for Phase II Progress Review: September 1, 2002

FIGURE 4.3. Doug's Treatment Plan.

Time	Planned Activities (including Sleep)	Anticipated Pleasure/ Sleep Quality (0–100)	Actual Activities & Sleep Schedule	Actual Pleasure/ Sleep Quality (0–100)
6 A.M.				
7 A.M.				
8 A.M.				
9 A.M.				
10 A.M.				
11 A.M.				
12 P.M.				
1 P.M.				
2 P.M.				
3 P.M.				
4 P.M.				
5 P.M.				
6 P.M.				
7 P.M.				
8 P.M.				
9 P.M.				
10 P.M.				
11 P.M.				
12 A.M.				
1 A.M.				
2–4 A.M.				
4–6 A.M.				

FIGURE 4.4. Log of Daily Activities and Sleep.

Urge to Drink		Drinks		
Date and Time	Strength of Urge (1–7)	Date and Time	Type	How Much

FIGURE 4.5. Diary of Urges and Drinks.

(see Appendix for information about how to obtain the Dyadic Adjustment Scale). Doug made reasonable progress in the second phase of treatment. He cut down his drinking and maintained a stable mood. His marital satisfaction did not improve significantly, so in the third phase of treatment, Doug and his wife entered couple therapy.

ESTABLISHING A MEASUREMENT PLAN

The first thing to consider in developing the measurement plan is how the data will be used. The therapist also has to think about how much change to expect (and how quickly), because this will determine how often the measures are collected. We generally establish an assessment plan at the beginning of treatment, but the plan often changes as the client moves through different phases of treatment. These changes occur for all the same reasons that the focus of treatment changes: New problems are discovered, crises develop, and some problems are resolved. In this section, we discuss these and other factors to keep in mind when planning a measurement strategy.

How Do I Want to Use the Data?

Perhaps the most important decision in designing a measurement plan is determining what will be done with the data once they are collected. Knowing how the information will be used can help to pinpoint the necessary domains to measure. As discussed in Chapter 3, each phase of treatment should include measures that reflect progress toward the aims addressed in the intervention for that phase. However, we often include some brief measurement of aspects of the client's symptoms or functioning that we do not plan to directly address at that time.

For example, Calvin sought treatment for his problems with compulsive behaviors (e.g., organizing his extensive collection of teapots, walking over the same ground repeatedly until it felt "just right") and an inability to establish close relationships. He also described frequent episodes of binge eating, with occasional regurgitation. Because he reported a past history of eating disordered behavior and some obsessive ideation related to his body image, the therapist asked Calvin to complete the Bulimia Test—Revised (BULIT-R; Thelen, Farmer, Wonderlich, & Simi, 1991), a 28-item, multiple choice, self-report scale used for measuring the severity of bulimic symptoms (see Appendix).

The therapist also included self-monitoring of binge eating and purging in her assessment plan, even though she did not intend to intervene directly during the limited number of sessions with Calvin. In this case, she did not expect to see change in the binge eating, but she wanted more information to support her conceptualization of the relationship between the eating problems and the compulsive behavior, and to provide more informed recommendations for future treatment. Furthermore, the results of the self-monitoring reassured the therapist that she was correct to view these problems as less serious than Calvin's compulsive behavior, which she assessed with the Yale–Brown Obsessive Compulsive Scale (Y-BOCS; Goodman et al., 1989; see Appendix).

The measurement plan for Calvin focused exclusively on symptoms, or *intra*personal issues (changes within the client). *Inter*personal functioning (involving the client's important relationships) and social role performance (functioning in occupational, family, and community roles) are often valuable areas for assessment (Lambert, 1994). In some cases, all three content domains (i.e., intrapersonal, interpersonal, social role performance) are assessed, but in many cases this would be excessive. At a minimum, the acute presenting problems should be tracked to gauge whether the intervention has been effective.

In a collaborative approach, the client and therapist may at times have different priorities about what problems should be monitored. For example, Jen was an adolescent client who sought treatment because her panic disorder interfered with school, work, and socializing. Although Jen endorsed the aim of reducing the frequency of panic attacks, she focused on minimizing the likelihood of an attack while she was with her new boyfriend, a possibility that particularly embarrassed her. The therapist wanted to keep a general record of panic attacks across situations to gauge the effectiveness of treatment, but Jen also wanted to monitor her embarrassment level with her boyfriend. Although the embarrassment was not a specific focus of the planned intervention, the therapist agreed to include this additional domain in self-monitoring because it was important to Jen.

How Frequently Should I Measure?

The general guideline for when to evaluate clients is *early* and *often*. Beginning the assessment process early is advisable, because it establishes a baseline from which to compare subsequent results. At least three data points are needed to see what is really going on (i.e., to see if the behavior is increasing, decreasing, or staying the same). Baseline data are often relatively easy to gather because clients and therapists are highly motivated at the outset. However, collecting substantive baseline data before beginning the intervention is an unheard-of luxury in most clinical settings. To improve the reliability of the baseline, we suggest using a measure of behavior that occurs relatively frequently (such as a sleep diary), so that daily, or even hourly, rather than weekly measures can be obtained. Retrospective reporting can provide information about the client's functioning in the few weeks before treatment began. Although retrospective reports are often inaccurate, this information can still provide some sense of the pattern of functioning before direct monitoring begins. Some data are better than no data!

Assessments should also be *brief*. Although realistic expectations differ across settings, the standard wisdom is that therapists in full-time practice can count on using only about 5 minutes of evaluator time and 20 minutes of client time (outside of session). Note that longer evaluations are sometimes possible if good incentives are used, such as a strong rationale about the utility of the measures or a reward system for children. The goal is not to infringe on therapy time, so our own clients frequently fill out measures in the waiting room before a session or as homework between appointments.

Measuring progress too rarely may cause therapists to miss important information about patterns or triggers relevant to the problem behavior. For example, if mood were assessed only once a month, it would be difficult to observe variations in symptoms associated with interpersonal conflicts or holidays. On the other hand, measuring too frequently can be misleading because of reactivity. Usually, client reactivity occurs in a socially desirable direction, but we have occasionally seen cases in which clients became obsessive about the measure, so that it was counterproductive to their treatment. For example, a client with binge-eating disorder who was attempting to maintain weight loss became excessively focused on counting calories, with the consequence that it increased her preoccupation with shape and weight, and made her more vulnerable to a binge episode. In our experience, this consequence of regular measurement is rare; it is a far more common problem to have insufficient assessment points.

How Much Change Do I Expect?

One aspect of treatment planning is development of a sense of how much change to expect before the next Progress Review. This expectation is based on many factors, including the nature of the problem, and the client's personality and life circumstances. Problems that are not expected to change, because they are not the focus of that particular treatment phase (e.g., frequency of arguments with spouse), may not be assessed on a regular basis unless the problem is serious (e.g., the arguments sometimes turn violent). As another example, a clinician treating a severely depressed client may expect a reduction in *symptoms* before the first review date, but she may hold little hope of a change in level of *functioning* by that date given the severity of depression at the outset. Nevertheless, because both magnitude of change and functioning level are critical, she may choose to measure both.

Should I Include Significant Others in the Assessment?

Despite the importance of the client's perspective, self-report can at times be misleading or insufficient on its own. Some clinical problems are frequently characterized by biased self-report, including eating disorders, substance abuse, and spousal abuse. In these cases, some other form of assessment is needed to supplement the self-report. Even in the absence of concerns about inaccurate or dishonest reporting, evaluating how other people see the client can increase confidence in the assessment. Getting the perspective of others also helps to establish the stability of the client's functioning across situations. For example, children may not be able to provide enough information about their aggressive behavior to be useful for treatment planning, but a report from parents or teachers regarding playground behavior can establish important triggers and environmental contingencies. Also, therapists can feel more confident about terminating treatment if multiple informers provide corroborating evidence that aggression has been reduced.

Most assessment tools for children include versions for parent and teacher reports in addition to the child report. These instruments generally must be purchased, but most of them have been carefully developed to maximize reliability and validity; all include age-appropriate norms. Some of the most common measures include the Child Behavior Checklist (to assess competencies and behavioral/emotional problems for children and young adults), Conners' Rating Scales—Revised (to assess attention-deficit/hyperactivity disorder and oppositional behavior among children and adolescents), the Behavior Assessment System for Children (to assess symptoms including depression and anxiety), and the Children's Depression Inventory (a self-report scale of depression for children ages 7–17) (see Appendix for information about how to obtain these assessment tools).

Should I Use Specific or General Measures?

Various measures target different levels of analysis, often involving a trade-off. Very specific information, such as how frequently a client with body dysmorphic disorder uses a mirror to shave, can be critical for treatment planning. These idiographic measures target unique problems experienced as troublesome by specific clients and may be more sensitive to change over the course of treatment. These highly tailored measures do have a downside. They usually cannot be applied across different clients or therapists, and they may not reflect meaningful improvement in the client's life. For example, assessing the frequency of eye contact during role plays during treatment may not be a good proxy for improvement on social skills, because eye contact is only one element of the skills required for positive social interactions. In contrast, more general information, such as global symptoms or role functioning, is applicable to a wider range of client problems but is often not as helpful for planning treatment with a particular client. In addition, these global measures can be less sensitive to changes related to specific client goals.

Global Measures

Some clinicians are interested in collecting information about overall distress or functioning. Global measures usually have norms, so that a client can be compared to a normative sample. Indeed, some insurance companies request such comparative information. Clients also occasionally request comparative information, and parents may request normative information about their child. Global measures are also useful for clinicians who want to compare progress across clients. We have used this strategy when conducting brief group therapy. Finally, global measures are essential for those therapists who want to keep track of overall improvement rates among clients in their caseload; some therapists are simply curious about this; others provide this information to interested clients during the initial evaluation and treatment planning stage.

When feasible, we recommend the use of at least one global measure that applies to every client. Global measures of client status, such as wide-ranging symptom measures and indicators of client functioning, are commonly available. We describe several such measures below.

The Behavior and Symptom Identification Scale (BASIS-32; Eisen, Dill, & Grob, 1994), a comprehensive measure of symptoms and functioning, assesses domains ranging from role responsibilities and relationships to impulsivity and suicidality. See *http://www.basis-32.org* for a copy of the scale and more information. The BASIS-32 is internally consistent and has shown good test–retest reliability. The scores are related to objective indicators such as rehospitalization and employment status. The subscales (relation to self and others, daily living and role functioning, depression and anxiety, impulsive and addictive behavior, and psychosis) correspond reasonably well to patient diagnoses, although the subscales tend to be correlated.

For settings that serve more severely ill clients, the Brief Psychiatric Rating Scale (BPRS; Overall & Gorham, 1962) is a good option. Originally developed with inpatient samples, the BPRS is a clinician-rated scale that assesses domains of functioning ranging from anxiety and emotional withdrawal to hallucinatory behavior and unusual thought content. The scale relies on a combination of self-report from the client and observations by the clinician, and takes 20–30 minutes to complete. Items for the BPRS are available in the Appendix; please see Rhoades and Overall (1988) for helpful sample questions to guide the interviewer, because each item is associated with a definition that is necessary for the rating. The BPRS has good interrater reliability and impressive indicators of validity. In addition, it is sensitive to treatment change and has shown adequate cross-cultural reliability (Dingemans, Winter, Bleeker, & Rathod, 1983).

The Global Assessment of Functioning scale is a one-item scale presented as Axis V in the fourth edition of the *Diagnostic and Statistical Manual of Mental Disorders* (DSM-IV; American Psychiatric Association, 1994). The clinician rates the item on the basis of overall psychosocial functioning, including role functioning and symptom severity. Single-item scales often have problems with reliability, but this is a readily available option for those settings with severe time and cost restrictions.

Other commonly used global measures are available for a fee; information about how to obtain these measures is included in the Appendix. (Please note that we do not have a financial stake in any of these measures or the companies that provide them.) The Medical Outcomes Survey Short Form (McHorney, Ware, & Raczek, 1993; Ware & Sherbourne, 1992), which is now called the RAND 36-Item Health Status Inventory, assesses physical and mental aspects of overall health in objective and relatively concrete terms, including indicators such as number of workdays missed, frequency of visits to the family physician, or ability to engage fully in family and home responsibilities. In addition to the popular 36-item version, a 12-item version is also available that takes about 2 minutes to complete. Both versions have representative, age-structured norms for clients 18–65 years of age.

The Brief Symptom Inventory (BSI; Derogatis & Melisaratos, 1983) provides questions about frequently encountered physical and emotional complaints such as nervousness, headaches, insomnia, and worry. The BSI is a briefer version of the popular Symptom Checklist-90—Revised (SCL-90-R), including the same nine symptom dimensions (somatization, obsessive–compulsive, interpersonal sensitivity, depression, anxiety, hostility, phobic anxiety, paranoid ideation, and psychoticism). Because the correlations between the BSI and SCL-90-R are very high, the briefer version may be more cost-effective.

In addition, one can consider using the Social Adjustment Scale—Self-Report (SAS-SR; Weissman & Bothwell, 1976). Although the SAS-SR takes 15–20 minutes to complete, it has been used in a wide variety of populations to assess the ability of adults to adapt and to be satisfied with their social roles.

Third-party payers and program evaluators are sometimes interested in assessing client satisfaction. Client satisfaction measures can address some important questions, particularly those related to clinic administration and positive feelings toward the therapy process, but they do not usually provide information useful for treatment planning. Clients may report satisfaction with the treatment if they feel that the therapist made a good-faith effort, whether or not they made progress on their initial complaints. In addition, clients may similarly feel reluctant to indicate poor satisfaction with the treatment due to their positive regard for therapists. Thus, client satisfaction measures can be difficult to interpret from the perspective of goal attainment.

Measures designed to assess client satisfaction include the Service Satisfaction Scale (Greenfield & Attkisson, 1989) and the SHARP Consumer Satisfaction Scales (Tanner, 1982; Tanner & Stacey, 1985). Information about how to obtain these measures is included in the Appendix.

Problem-Specific Measures

Because global measures typically do not guide treatment planning for individual clients as well as idiographic measures, we advise adding problem-specific measures even when a client satisfaction or other global measurement system is already in place. A literature review reveals a wealth of measures that can be used to track specific problems over the course of treatment. Therapy outcome studies are a good place to start; these articles provide references for obtaining the measures used to evaluate specific symptoms that characterize a given diagnostic category.

Keri was a 32-year-old client referred with a diagnosis of borderline personality disorder. Her therapist recognized that therapy would likely go through several phases, so he decided to administer the BASIS-32 (described earlier) on a monthly basis as an overall indicator of functioning. Additional measures were obviously called for, but the therapist did not necessarily expect to see changes in Keri's primary diagnosis. For that reason, he did not administer a measure designed to assess borderline personality features (e.g., the Borderline Personality Inventory; Falk, 1999). Instead, he prioritized Keri's depressive symptoms and overall self-esteem as specific targets of change during the first phase of treatment. Accordingly, in addition to the BASIS-32, Keri completed the BDI on a weekly basis and the Rosenberg Self-Esteem Scale (Rosenberg, 1962; see Appendix) every other week.

As an example of very different problems, Les, a 44-year-old man, had struggled with schizophrenia for his entire adult life. In the community mental health center where Les was treated, the BPRS (described earlier) was used with most clients with chronic mental illness. Les had experienced auditory hallucinations throughout the course of his illness, but the severity of these symptoms varied over time. In addition, Les had an ongoing delusion that his consumption of food and water, as well as his use of personal hygiene products such as toothpaste, toilet paper, and soap, had a negative impact on other people. For example, Les believed that if he drank too much water during the day, he would make his mother ill.

Because of the impact of these delusions on his basic functioning, Les's social worker wanted more specific information about the severity of his psychotic symptoms than the BPRS provides and specifically assessed important aspects of his hallucinations and delusions using the Psychotic Symptom Rating Scales (PSYRATS; see Appendix; Haddock, McCarron, Tarrier, & Faragher, 1999) during her interviews with him. The clinician also asked Les to monitor the amount of water and number of meals he consumed each day, and she created behavioral schedules that included a scripted personal hygiene routine.

Different measurement modalities provide unique information useful for treatment planning. *Self-report questionnaires* are the most common method of measurement. Although these measures are not perfect (sometimes being subject to response bias and social desirability effects), self-report is the most direct assessment of the client's cognitive and emotional experiences. In contrast, *psychophysiological mea-sures* are usually less prone to reactivity, but practicing clinicians outside of behavioral medicine rarely use them, because the equip-ment is expensive (with the exception of scales for weighing clients with eating disorders). Nonetheless, technological advances may make this important source of information more accessible to the average cli-nician. For example, inexpensive, easy-to-use, portable heart rate mon-itors are now commonly available.

Self-monitoring is almost always useful whenever the problem be-havior involves a discrete behavior such as arguments, homework, hair pulling, social activities, or eating. Therapists devise these self-monitoring forms to correspond to the information required for assess-ment. For example, in a smoking cessation treatment, a client's moni-toring form can be used to count the number of cigarettes smoked, as well as to identify triggers for smoking and cravings (e.g., interper-sonal conflict and negative affect). See Figure 4.6 for a sample cigarette self-monitoring form, filled out by one of our clients.

One challenge with self-monitoring is that the client first needs to notice the behavior or response before she or he can record it. Not sur-prisingly, this requires some vigilance and motivation, so it is impor-tant to consider strategies to enhance compliance and accuracy (see Hayes et al., 1999). For example, *discussing potential barriers* to monitor-ing often identifies problems that can be addressed before they inter-fere with the task. One of our clients, Connie, wanted to improve her time management skills and reduce the number of times she missed appointments or confused the time of meetings. Her therapist sug-gested that she check her electronic organizer each day to tally the number of successfully attended meetings versus those she missed or at which she arrived late. However, when the therapist asked Connie whether she foresaw any difficulties with this assignment, she noted that she regularly misplaced her organizer and that this was a key part of the original problem.

Connie and her therapist then considered how to *make the monitor-ing feasible*. Connie decided she would buy a basket that she would keep at her front door, where she could drop her keys and organizer when she arrived home. Another step involved *provision of training* in the self-monitoring task; during a session, Connie's therapist helped her use the previous day's entries from the organizer to create a chart of successful versus missed appointments. Finally, to help Connie rec-ognize the value of the data collected from the task and to help main-tain motivation, the therapist provided *reinforcement for collection of ac-*

Date & Time	Trigger (situation, thoughts, feelings)	Craving Strength (1–7)	# of Cigarettes Smoked
7/16 10 A.M.	Boss was critical of me, thought = I'm a loser, feeling = sad	6	1
Noon	Lunch break, thought = everyone is smoking now, feeling = tired	4	0
4 P.M.	Fight with coworker, thought = I'm all alone, feeling = angry	7	2

FIGURE 4.6. Self-Monitoring of Cigarette Craving and Smoking.

curate data at the beginning of each session through verbal praise and by using the results of the self-monitoring during the session.

Self-monitoring can take many forms, including diaries (e.g., food or panic attack records; see Figures 4.2 and 4.7), frequency counts (e.g., occurrence of obsessions or number of social engagements), or duration of events (e.g., length of anger outbursts or time spent compulsively washing). Simply by recording the occurrence of an event, positive behaviors typically increase in frequency while undesirable behaviors decrease (Cavior & Marabotto, 1976; Sieck & McFall, 1976). Although this raises some concern about the accuracy of self-monitoring data, in this case, the measurement process not only provides valuable information for treatment planning but also promotes treatment goals.

Direct observation can occur within the therapy setting, including "molar" or global rating scales of functioning or "molecular" ratings of specific behaviors (e.g., such as the frequency that a person with tapping rituals knocks on the table during a session). It is also possible to systematically observe naturally occurring behaviors in therapeutic settings (e.g., number of client interruptions during a session) or behaviors in a role-play situation (e.g., frequency of stuttering during a simulated job interview). Direct observation can also be conducted in natural environments by significant others, clinic staff, or mechanical recording devices.

Date	Intensity of attack (1–7)	Situation	Thoughts	Duration of Attack
11/2	3	Leaving for school	I can't cope.	15 min
11/2	6	Teacher called on me	I'm embarrassing myself.	5 min

FIGURE 4.7. Panic Attack Record.

Can I Create Measures from Scratch?

Whether to use an existing measure or create one specifically for a given client sometimes poses a dilemma. In general, existing measures are preferred because they have been carefully constructed to be reliable (i.e., repeated administrations of the measure yield the same result) and valid (i.e., they measure what they are purported to measure). Thus, use of an existing instrument permits confidence in the psychometric properties of the measure, including (sometimes) the availability of norms to which the client's score can be compared. On the other hand, there may be times when no published scale is available for a particular problem that needs to be monitored. In this case, practitioners may choose to develop their own measure tailored to particular clients.

We recommend first doing a search of the literature and measurement compendia to avoid "recreating the wheel." Figure 4.8 presents an idiographic measure designed for a client, Jesse, in which the therapist wanted to monitor changes in particular communication skills that either promoted or diminished Jesse's assertive responding with her husband Bob. No obvious measure was available to address the specificity of this assessment, because general measures of assertiveness did not reflect this focused domain. Accordingly, the therapist created her own list of assertiveness skills relevant to positive interactions within Jesse's marriage.

Each week, the therapist gave Jesse a new checklist to keep in her purse. Whenever Jesse had a disagreement with Bob, she would tally the number of positive and negative communication responses she believed she had used. Ideally, Bob could have provided similar ratings of Jesse's behaviors during their fights to corroborate her report, but he was not interested in participating in the therapy. At first, Jesse found it difficult to distinguish between the different types of responses, because she had been in the habit of making very global evaluations of each interaction as either "good" or "bad." To help her recognize specific behaviors, Jesse's therapist asked her to generate examples of the different categories from her own interactions with Bob, such as complaining about a headache during an argument to generate pity and evade answering an accusation.

Ultimately, Jesse was able to use the monitoring form to record marital interactions and to remind herself of her specific aims. Each week, Jesse's therapist reviewed the form with her and noted any negative behaviors that appeared to interfere frequently in her discussions

Positive Response Styles	# Times	Negative Response Styles	# Times
Express feelings calmly		Insult Bob	
Express feelings directly		Make threats	
Describe behavior objectively		Whine or use an apologetic voice	
Ask for change that is reasonable		Ignore Bob	
Reinforce positive responses		Laugh off Bob's response	
Consider my rights and goals		Make accusations	
Consider Bob's rights/goals		Delay unfairly	
Maintain direct eye contact		Quibble/bicker	
Speak clearly		Play to or for self-pity	
Listen carefully to Bob		Deny unfairly	
Acknowledge Bob's position		Overemphasize past difficulties	
Attempt to compromise		Stay quiet/not speak up	
Repeat request if initially ignored		Give up after only one attempt	
Content-to-process shift		Be overly demanding	
Defuse situation		Present issues in black-and-white terms	
Assertive delay (wait until calm)		Take the bait in front of the kids	
Assertive agreement		Ignore positive feedback	
Assertive inquiry		Jump to negative conclusions	
Other:		Other:	
Comments (unusual events, etc.): _____			

FIGURE 4.8. Jesse's Assertive Responding Checklist.

with Bob. The therapist noted that on several occasions Jesse had laughed at Bob's anger (based on the number of marks on the monitoring form), which had only served to further escalate the disagreement. Jesse decided that her goal for the next week was to listen to her husband's position before responding. The monitoring form served as both a tool to track progress (by calculating the proportion of positive to negative responses each week) and a guide for Jesse to make positive changes.

What Do I Do When the Measures Disagree?

Incongruence across different sources of measurement is common. In fact, it is the norm rather than the exception in certain domains, such as anxiety disorders. Anxiety researchers debate the reasons why fear responses differ across measures (e.g., why someone whose heart is racing when confronted with a feared stimulus may show no avoidance). One suggestion is that different modalities of responding reflect distinct, albeit related, constructs. This hypothesis proposes that fear may be expressed in the realms of behavior, physiology, cognition, and affect, but that the pattern of response across these modalities varies depending on the person. Alternatively, others have proposed that the measures tap the same underlying construct, but that the incongruence is due to measurement error.

Depending on the context, measures that disagree can be used in different ways for treatment planning and evaluation. One strategy is to attend to the indicator with the poorest results to determine the focus of the next phase of treatment; that is, if a client who says she is not anxious is still avoiding, then the next treatment intervention can target avoidance behavior. The measures indicating the best performance (reduction in self-reported fear in this example) can be used as motivators to reinforce treatment progress. Thus, in the Progress Review with the client, consider emphasizing the measure that highlights positive change while using the index of poor progress to direct the next phase of the Treatment Plan.

Discrepancy between measures can also confirm or clarify the nature of the problem for which the client seeks therapy. For example, disagreement on measures of marital satisfaction may be the reason spouses need a mediator who can point out discrepancies and highlight similarities across ratings. In other cases, discrepant measures lead the therapist to doubt the accuracy of one of the measures rather than considering them as alternate, equally valid pieces of data. In this case, O'Leary and Wilson (1987) recommend several strategies to help reduce discrepancies across raters or measures in which a unified result was expected. One helpful strategy is to make sure that interview questions are structured in comparable terms when asking multiple people the same question. For example, ask both a parent and teacher, "How frequently does John hit another child?" rather than asking one about hitting and the other how often John gets angry. Consistency in the question increases the chances that the two raters will interpret the question in the same way. In addition, increased congruence and accuracy can be obtained by measuring easily quantifiable current events (such as grades, frequency of arrests, time to rehospitalization) that are relatively objective and require minimal inference.

CASE STUDY: GROUP TREATMENT FOR SOCIAL PHOBIA

To illustrate the direct application of outcome data to treatment planning, we describe the measurement plan and Progress Review for a social phobia group we conducted. Several clients with social phobia were scheduled to participate in a group treatment that was initially contracted for 12 sessions. Mitch, a 35-year-old law student who was completing his second year and applying for clerkships, had generalized social phobia, and his primary concerns were dating and evaluative situations with other law students and professors. Madeleine, a 36-year-old website designer with long-standing social phobia exacerbated by her recent relocation, had almost no social contacts and was experiencing moderate depression. Solana, a 27-year-old guidance counselor whose family emigrated from a Near Eastern country when she was a child, was primarily concerned about formal social situations, such as entertaining at home, but she also avoided informal gatherings such as joining her coworkers for lunch. Layne, a 29-year-old man engaged to be married the following summer, experienced intense anxiety whenever he was the focus of attention. His job required routine presentations, but he had been putting them off and was several months behind. Furthermore, he worried intensely about the social demands of his upcoming wedding. Finally, Letitia, a 28-year-old graduate student in music composition, was unable to speak in her classes. Generalized social phobia prevented her from dating and hampered her efforts to seek mentoring and guidance in graduate school, and to break into a career in music.

What to Measure?

Because the group was composed of people with fairly similar problems (generalized social phobia), the therapists decided to forego global measures in favor of those specific to the presenting problem. The only exception was the decision to include the Beck Depression Inventory (BDI) given that several group members were experiencing depressive symptoms.

Clients with social phobia often anticipate more anxiety for an upcoming social interaction than they experience when actually in the situation. Because of this problem, the therapists decided to conduct a behavioral assessment, in addition to self-report, involving participation in two brief, standardized social situations (an impromptu speech in front of an audience and a conversation with a stranger). Indicators of the severity of social phobia from this assessment included clients' self-rated anxiety and social performance, audience (and conversation partner) ratings of anxious appearance and social performance, and degree of avoidance or escape (operationalized as number of minutes spent in each situation).

More generalized social anxiety was measured with the Social Phobia Anxiety Inventory (SPAI), a self-report measure that covers a wide range of social situations. (See the Appendix for information on obtaining the SPAI.) Both the BDI and the SPAI have published norms and good reliability and validity profiles, and the behavioral assessment is widely used in research on social phobia. Finally, the group therapists conducted an unstructured interview with clients to elicit their opinions regarding the parameters and severity of their primary problems.

How and When to Measure?

The behavioral assessment has the advantage of being conducted by an independent evaluator (in order to eliminate the artifact of the therapists' calming presence). However, this assessment is expensive in terms of staffing, so it can be used only rarely. The SPAI and BDI, much less expensive measures, can be used more frequently. Accordingly, the therapists decided to use a behavioral assessment (with administrative staff members and graduate students as assistants) and the unstructured individual interview before the group began and again at the conclusion of the treatment. Clients completed the SPAI and BDI once a month. After 12 weeks of treatment, the therapists evaluated progress and decided whether to continue within the same treatment phase, begin a new phase, or terminate therapy.

Results demonstrated the value of multimodal assessment, because the findings for several clients surprised the therapists. Before the final assessment, the therapists believed Mitch had made good progress on his anxiety related to his role as a law student, but they were concerned that he still maintained extremely rigid rules about social behavior (such as beginning casual conversations with women). Nevertheless, they did not anticipate that Mitch would continue in therapy, because he did not appear to share the therapists' view of this problem. Mitch's formal evaluation was very informative. His SPAI and BDI showed good improvement, supporting the therapists' initial opinion. His performance in the behavioral assessment was extremely good, with only moderate anxiety during a very skillful performance. The independent evaluator gave him explicit feedback about the high quality of his performance, but in a meeting with the therapists immediately afterward, Mitch was despondent. He stated that he had "completely bombed" the speech and role-play conversation. Furthermore, Mitch agreed with the therapists about the goal of being less rigid in interactions with women. They decided together on Phase II treatment goals, which would be addressed in individual treatment.

During group sessions, Madeleine had such a withdrawn presence that the therapists believed she was quite depressed. They had been monitoring her monthly BDI scores and encouraged her to consider simultaneous individual treatment for depression. They did not believe she had made much progress on her social phobia. At the 12-week assessment point, Madeleine showed lower anxiety and less avoidance in her behavioral assessment, and her SPAI score showed good improvement. Her BDI score was 13, indicating relatively mild depression, which was somewhat of a surprise to the therapists. Nevertheless, in her interview with the therapists, Madeleine expressed an interest in continuing treatment, with the aims of decreasing depression, improving her contentious relationship with her husband, and managing her combativeness during times of anger.

Solana's formal evaluation was the most unexpected of all the group members. The therapists perceived Solana to be doing quite well and were prepared to terminate treatment with her. At most, they planned to recommend a few booster sessions to review material covered in the group. Solana showed good improvement in the behavioral assessment, and her BDI continued to show extremely low levels of depression. However, Solana's SPAI scores had not improved at all. Because this measure has been established as quite sensitive to treatment change, the therapists recommended continued work on social phobia, broadening the focus to the wide variety of situations Solana still avoided.

Layne showed the most improvement in his behavioral assessment, which was consistent with the therapists' impressions. Before treatment, Layne was not even able to begin his speech; he broke down in tears when he faced the audience. At the 12-week assessment point, Layne completed both tasks with only moderate anxiety, and his social skills were well within the normal range. His SPAI and BDI scores showed good improvement. The therapists recommended that he end therapy at this point, reminding him that he might wish to return in the early autumn for two or three sessions to help him cope with the social performance aspects of the wedding.

Finally, Letitia demonstrated good progress in terms of being able to accomplish goals such as speaking in class, consulting with professors, and networking with other graduate students. Her behavioral assessment showed good progress on anxiety and avoidance, and her SPAI showed good improvement. However, Letitia's BDI scores revealed that she was moderately depressed. In reviewing these results together, Letitia and the therapists planned for Phase II to involve individual treatment for depression.

This lengthy case example illustrates the value of formal assessment and Progress Review. The two group therapists had discussed each client after every session and carefully charted their observations of improvement. Furthermore, they had asked clients to agree to between-session social activities to promote the goals of treatment, and they discussed these activities at the beginning of each session. Accordingly, they felt they knew the clients fairly well and had made tentative disposition plans for each. Most of these plans were changed when the therapists reviewed the results of the formal evaluation, including self-report questionnaires and behavioral assessment. What became clear was that the information on client status that arises naturally during a session is not a complete picture of symptoms or functioning, even though it may seem comprehensive at the time.

SHORTCUTS FOR THE BUSY CLINICIAN

Measurement during therapy is a worthwhile but challenging activity. In Table 4.2, we summarize some of the challenges commonly encountered in developing a measurement plan and suggest corresponding strategies to guide the selection and implementation of measures in clinical practice.

We have assembled a resource list to provide help in more easily accessing and using measures. Although not exhaustive, the following list of concrete suggestions for how to obtain assessment tools focuses on measures of clinically relevant problems, such as assessments of symptoms, behavior, and functioning that are expected to be responsive to therapeutic interventions. Accordingly, it does not include achievement tests, personality assessment, or neuropsychiatric tests. We have incorporated a broad range of biopsychosocial constructs as aids in treatment planning and reviewing progress, with an emphasis on measures likely to show change in response to psychotherapy.

TABLE 4.2. Strategies to Guide Ongoing Measurement of Treatment Progress

Challenge	Strategy
Ensure that measures will be useful.	Determine in advance what you will do with the data once you collect it, and consider what information is needed for treatment planning or for other interested parties, such as third-party payers.
Measure change on multiple levels.	Incorporate both global and specific measures to assess change in problematic symptoms as well as general functioning.
Make broad treatment goals specific.	State problems in specific terms, so that vague goals can be made concrete and quantifiable, enabling more direct measurement.
Gather data beyond treatment outcome variables.	Consider the value of assessing treatment process variables, client satisfaction, and motivation or readiness to change.
Have multiple sources for assessment.	Look for congruence across client reports and information provided by trained observers, relevant others, the therapist, and institutional ratings.
Use measures for treatment planning even when they disagree.	Consider why the incongruence is occurring (different rates of change, inaccurate reporting, etc.) and use this information for treatment planning.
Take advantage of multiple methods of measurement.	Use a variety of methodologies, such as self-report, self-monitoring, psychophysiological, and direct observation, to increase confidence in interpretations of progress.
Combine existing and idiographic measures.	Benefit from the specificity of idiographic measures, but combine them with measures that have norms and established psychometric properties.
Make assessment feasible and cost-effective.	Measure early and often by choosing measures that are not only brief and easy to use but also reliable and valid.
Search for culturally sensitive instruments.	Strive for "diversity competency" by being scientifically minded and searching for measures designed for the particular client population.

Websites

The Science Directorate of the American Psychological Association website (*http://www.apa.org/science/findingtests.pdf*) has extensive information about how to locate and access published and unpublished psychological tests and measures. In addition, the site addresses frequently asked questions about finding tests and using them properly. The Directorate neither sells nor endorses testing instruments, but it does provide guidance in using available resources to find psychological tests.

The ERIC/AE website (*http://ericae.net*) describes itself as a clearinghouse for assessment, evaluation, and research information, and is particularly focused on resources for educational assessment. In addition, the site contains the ERIC/AE Test Locator, a searchable database of test descriptions with over 10,000 entries. The site also contains the Buros/ERIC Test Publisher Directory, which provides access to the names and addresses of over 900 major commercial test publishers.

Databases

These databases can be used by individuals for a fee, but they are commonly available through libraries. Visit each website to learn more about access to each specific database. Generally, using a broad search engine and entering the title of the database will quickly direct the user to an entry site.

PsycINFO (*http://www.apa.org/psycinfo/*) provides information about psychological research in general, but it can also serve as a useful starting point to locate references for particular measures. It covers materials from 1967 to the present and is updated frequently. In thinking about developing a treatment plan, this is also a good place to search for clinical outcome trials to evaluate the effectiveness of a particular therapeutic approach with various client populations. This resource is available at most university libraries, but individuals can also arrange to use the database for a fee.

Health and Psychosocial Instruments (HAPI) provides information on measurement instruments (i.e., questionnaires, interview schedules, checklists, index measures, coding schemes/manuals, rating scales, projective techniques, vignettes/scenarios, tests) in the health fields, psychosocial sciences, and organizational behavior. See their website at *http://www.library.mcgill.ca/peruse/healthpsychosocial.htm*. This database searches for primary or secondary source material, or both. It covers materials from 1985 forward, along with many earlier measures, and is updated every few months.

Books

Educational Measurement, 3rd edition, Phoenix, AZ: Oryx Press, 1993. Sponsored jointly by the National Council on Measurement in Education and the American Council on Education, this work covers general principles in educational measurement, pragmatic applications, and test construction.

A Guide to 85 Tests for Special Education, Belmont, MA: Fearon Education, 1990. This guide includes assessments related to academic performance, perception, memory and visual–motor skills, speech and language, bilingualism, gross and fine motor coordination, and general intelligence tests and scales.

Handbook of Family Measurement Techniques, Newbury Park, CA: Sage, 1990. This handbook covers nearly 1,000 instruments arranged by five primary categories: interaction within families, intimacy and family values, parenthood, roles and power, and adjustment. It also provides information on availability, variables measured and the type of instrument, short descriptions, sample items, comments, and article references and reviews, and includes indexes by author, title, and subject classification.

Handbook of Psychiatric Measures, Washington, DC: American Psychiatric Association, 2000. Developed by the American Psychiatric Association Task Force for the Handbook of Psychiatric Measures, the handbook includes a compendium of rating scales and measures useful for assessment of mental illnesses, as well as a CD-ROM that includes copies of 108 measures discussed in the handbook.

Handbook of Psychological Assessment, 2nd edition, New York: Wiley, 1990. Strategies for assessment (interviewing, observing, testing) and general overviews of the seven most frequently used tests are included in this handbook, which also gives guidelines for psychological report writing and formatting, and provides sample reports.

Major Psychological Assessment Instruments, 2nd edition, Boston: Allyn & Bacon, 1996. This book provides in-depth descriptions and interpretations of the most widely used psychological assessments.

Measures for Clinical Practice: A Sourcebook, 3rd edition, 2 volumes, New York: Free Press, 2000. This popular collection of short, easily scored measures from Corcoran and Fischer is a practical tool. The first volume includes measures for use with couples, families, and children, and the second has measures appropriate for assessing therapy with adults outside the family context. They cover most problems seen in clinical practice and introduce basic principles of measurement and an overview of different types of measures.

The Mental Measurements Yearbooks, Highland Park, NJ: Gryphon Press/Buros Institute of Mental Measurements, 1938 to present. These well-known yearbooks list and describe commercially published tests produced or revised in English. They include critical reviews of tests and references to relevant publications, and provide useful indexes including title, acronym, and classified subject.

Sex and Gender Issues: A Handbook of Tests and Measures, New York: Greenwood Press, 1990. This useful book describes nearly 200 scales covering topics such as eating disorders, pregnancy and childbirth, and sexuality. It also provides sample items, variables measured, descriptions, administration, scoring techniques, reliability and validity, availability, and references.

Tests: A Comprehensive Reference for Assessments in Psychology, Education and Business, 2nd edition, Kansas City, MO: Test Corporation of America, 1986. This resource lists and describes 3,500 tests in English and identifies the publisher or distributor of each. A companion volume, *Test Critiques,* discusses practical applications and contains critical reviews.

Tests in Print, Lincoln, NE: Buros Institute of Mental Measurements, 1961 to present. This scaled-down version of the *Mental Measurements Yearbooks* lists commercially published tests and references to publications on the tests, but without the critical reviews. Four indexes include title, classified subject, publishers, and author. Newer editions contain cross-references to earlier editions of this work and to the previous *Mental Measurements Yearbooks.*

CHAPTER 5

ILLUSTRATING PROGRESS THROUGH GRAPHING

In the preceding chapters, we described how to produce the Problem List and outline the initial phase of the Treatment Plan (including aims, strategies, and measures). Graphing the results of ongoing measurement is easy to do and facilitates interpretation of the measures, as well as communication of the results to the client and others. In this chapter, we describe how to set up a simple system for managing and visually inspecting the information collected throughout the measurement process. Whereas here we focus on graphing, in Chapter 6 we focus on regularly scheduled reviews to refine and direct the Treatment Plan.

The frequency of measurement partly determines when to inspect the data visually. For a problem monitored daily, the results can be graphed right from the first week. If the client completes a questionnaire on a weekly basis, it may be preferable to continue measurement for several weeks before graphing it. As we discussed in Chapter 4, the frequency of measurement depends on how often the problem occurs, as well as on some considerations related to the assessment tool (e.g., cost). In order for the assessment results to be maximally useful for treatment planning, we suggest using some types of measurement that occur relatively frequently. In fact, we often chart assessment results in the few minutes it takes to write progress notes from each session. Readily accessible computer spreadsheet programs aid in this process (e.g., Microsoft Excel, described later), although if computer access is limited, creating graphs by hand is a convenient, equally informative option. Although the graphs may look complicated at first glance, they can be created fairly quickly.

WHY GRAPH?: RATIONALE FOR VISUAL INSPECTION OF THE DATA

Graphing client data makes it easier to follow a client's progress. Although it takes a little time to transfer the data from the session or homework assignment to a graph, multiple benefits follow from the improved ability to monitor progress on an ongoing basis, generate detailed reports, and use visual aids to communicate with the client and others.

A Picture is Worth a Thousand Words

Graphs efficiently communicate a client's progress because they are both comprehensive and concise. Furthermore, visual representations often prove to be illuminating for clients. Although clients (and their therapists) may have a sense of whether things are getting better, worse, or staying the same, graphing provides a powerful illustration. Seeing progress represented on a graph feels like a reward for the time spent collecting the data. Graphing naturally summarizes data, dramatically reducing the time needed to conduct Progress Reviews. Visually evaluating the results of assessment is especially helpful when measuring multiple indicators of progress; that is, the client may show improvement on one measure while another remains the same. Recognizing the difference between measures can be helpful for directing future phases of treatment. For example, a client who has been self-monitoring his crying episodes may feel discouraged by the fact that he is crying just as often now as when he began treatment. However, if he has also shown a sizable drop in his score on a broader depression inventory, then the therapist may suspect that the treatment is having an impact on some depressive symptoms but not on others. The therapist and client may then decide to target more specifically the crying episodes in the subsequent phase of treatment.

Focusing on the Bigger Picture

Another advantage of graphing is that it can help the client to focus on the "big picture" even in the face of a few bad days. Rita, a teenager with bulimia nervosa, entered treatment in August and made great strides in reducing her frequency of bingeing and purging over the first month of treatment. In September, however, she experienced a surge in binge-eating episodes and compensatory purging. Rita was demoralized by this lapse, feeling that she had taken "10 steps backward," and that all of her earlier hard work had been negated. Even though the frequency of Rita's bingeing and purging decreased steadily over the next month, her negative mood persisted. She also began to doubt her abilities in school, labeling herself as an "utter failure." During a session in the sixth week of treatment, Rita's therapist showed her a graph of the frequency of her bingeing and purging episodes. Rita was surprised to see that her lapse had lasted for only 4 days and that this increase coincided with the start of her senior year of high school. Her therapist used the graphic display of symptoms to help Rita generate alternative explanations for the increase in bingeing and purging (i.e., increased stress) and to reassure herself that the lapse did not last as long as it had seemed. The graph helped to remotivate Rita for treatment and reminded her of the importance of taking a long-term perspective on her progress.

Mastery and Self-Efficacy

Enhancing self-efficacy may be an important aim of treatment for many clients. Self-efficacy, also called a sense of mastery, is the belief that one is competent and able to carry out actions with success (Bandura, 1977). Clients can gain a sense of mastery over at least some aspects of their problem(s) by setting achievable treatment goals and observing—even celebrating—progress toward those goals. Taking an active role in assessing treatment progress and prioritizing the next steps can also boost self-efficacy and the client's sense of ownership of the therapy process. In other words, being able to ask and answer the question "How well have I met my goals, and what changes can I make to promote future success?" is one way for clients to take a more active role in their own progress.

Most people need some standard against which to measure their performance, and having a basis for judgment appears to boost development of new skills (Bandura & Schunk, 1981). Graphing in the

PACC model provides clients with a yardstick to judge, in a safe and supportive environment, exactly how much progress they have made toward their aims. Graphs present the feedback in a concrete and meaningful way that increases the client's perceived reward, which may in turn increase commitment and adherence (Putnam et al., 1994).

Using Graphs to Develop Aims

When things are going well, a graph highlights progress toward goals, reinforcing commitment to the process. If no progress has been made or, indeed, if the client has become worse, then the therapist can help the client evaluate this information, plan changes in strategies, and set more realistic short-term goals. In our experience, graphing can be very useful in helping the client identify and come to terms with the domains of functioning that need additional work. For example, one widely used measure of depressive symptomatology is the Beck Depression Inventory (BDI). The psychiatrist working with Tovah, a 37-year-old woman suffering from posttraumatic stress disorder (PTSD), regularly administered the BDI to monitor Tovah's level of depression.

The overarching goal of treatment was to decrease the intensity of the flashbacks, nightmares, avoidance, and dissociation that Tovah had begun experiencing following an assault by a stranger. Tovah had difficulty in treatment from the start, however, reporting that she could not concentrate in session or stay focused on what she needed to do. Over the ensuing months, Tovah began to report that she was feeling "dizzy and shaky all the time," and that she felt "stabbing pain" in her stomach and in her eyes. Tovah had "absolutely no idea" where these symptoms originated. The psychiatrist was uncertain whether these symptoms were a result of somatization, physical illness, or some other psychosomatic process. In session, the psychiatrist asked Tovah about her medical history, as well as her eating and sleeping habits; She denied having a problem. Tovah claimed that her overall routine was the same as it always had been.

The psychiatrist examined Tovah's self-report data, including some of the individual items on the BDI. She discovered that Tovah's BDI indicated that she had been eating and sleeping "a lot less than usual" over the previous 2 months. She made a very simple graph of these data, noting when Tovah had begun endorsing physical complaints on the questionnaire. The graph demonstrated that Tovah's self-report of physical difficulty coincided with her report of changes in eating and sleeping habits. When Tovah saw this graph, she began to discuss the extent of her problems with eating and sleeping.

Tovah reported that she typically went to bed at midnight but watched TV until 4 or 5 A.M. and got up at 7 A.M. She also reported that the only meal she had been eating regularly was lunch; for breakfast, she had "a few cups of coffee," and she typically snacked on chips and soda, her "comfort foods," for dinner. Her report provided some hypotheses about why she felt dizzy and shaky (from too much caffeine and too little food), had pains in her eyes (from lack of sleep and excessive TV viewing), and pains in her stomach (from hunger). Reviewing these observations with Tovah led to a new phase of treatment. The focus was temporarily diverted from her PTSD symptoms to meal planning and sleep regulation.

Graphing can be particularly important for clients whose problems naturally wax and wane over time, because noting patterns of symptoms (even retrospectively) can help the practitioner to identify important behavior patterns and communicate with the client about them. For example, many clients with bipolar disorder find that they are better able to manage their illness if they identify time periods (e.g., summer vs. winter) and situational triggers (e.g., increased stress, loss of sleep) when they are most at risk for an exacerbation of manic or depressive symptoms.

Graphing can also be very useful for clients with chronic mental health problems. Peggy, a 33-year-old woman with a diagnosis of schizophrenia, lived in a supervised residence and held a part-time job, but she cycled in and out of inpatient and partial hospital settings. When at her best, Peggy could implement a number of cognitive strategies to bring the auditory hallucinations "under control." She reported receiving command hallucinations (e.g., to throw a chair, eat dirt, or pull out her hair) but sometimes was able to tell herself, "I don't need to listen to what they say; they are just voices in my head." When Peggy was not functioning as well, she acted impulsively, following the commands of the voices and causing a great deal of damage to both herself and her surroundings.

For almost 10 years, Peggy was unable to accept that "stressors" contributed to the instability of her functioning, despite the psychoeducation she had received from several members of her treatment team. One of the therapists began graphing Peggy's stress level over time, as indicated by her subjective ratings of stress, the amount of sleep she was getting, and the frequency with which she sought her parents' advice (an indicator to Peggy that she was feeling overwhelmed). On the basis of these graphs, Peggy saw clearly that increases in stress immediately preceded her psychotic breaks and inpatient hospitalizations. When this information was displayed in a graphic form, Peggy reported that she had a much better understanding of the relationship between her stress and functioning.

Communicating with Children and Significant Others

Graphs can be particularly useful when working with children. School-age children can assist in making simple graphs, which adds to the perceived value of the graph and teaches them to monitor their own progress. Depending on the age and cognitive abilities of the child, graphing can help him or her both to visualize progress and set future goals. Parents often express appreciation and renewed motivation when visually reviewing their child's progress. Many parents, focused on long-range goals, forget how far their child has come in treatment. A visual reminder of progress helps to focus parents (or teachers) on the child's positive behaviors. The same principle applies to adult clients, who may wish to share the results of their assessment with an employer or spouse, particularly if others have expressed uncertainty about what is being accomplished in therapy. Simple graphs tell a story even to those who are relatively unsophisticated or uneducated.

CREATING GRAPHS

Figure 5.1 reviews the steps involved in using graphs to evaluate the results of assessment and to help plan subsequent phases of treatment. As a part of the Treatment Plan for each phase, the PACC therapist establishes a plan for measurement of progress. We usually begin graphing right from the beginning by forming the structure for the graph (whether on paper or on computer) with a title and labeling the axes to correspond to the selected measures. If possible, we collect enough baseline data to look for stability in the measure, but we still collect baseline data even if time permits only one observation. As treatment proceeds, we enter the data as we go along—usually when preparing progress notes for each session. (This data entry step takes less than a minute once the basic structure of the graph is in place.) Other clinicians using the PACC system may choose a prearranged time (approximately once a month) to enter graphical data across all clients. At scheduled intervals, we review progress with the client and change to

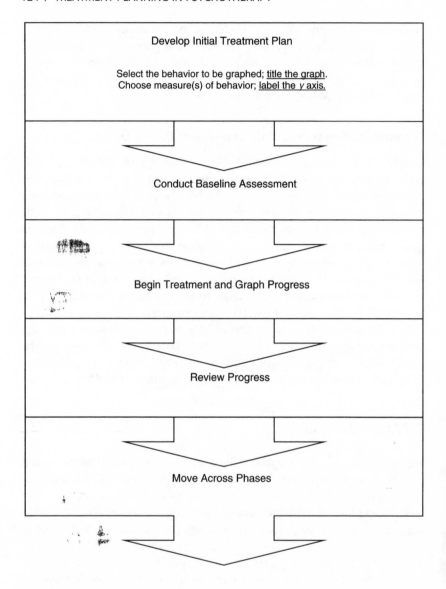

FIGURE 5.1. Schematic plan for measurement in the PACC system.

a new phase (marked on the graph) when appropriate. Of course, if the problem has resolved sufficiently that the new phase will address completely different problems, we are likely to end the original graph and begin a new one. In the next sections, we discuss the baseline evaluation in more detail before providing some tips on computer-based graphing.

Conducting the Baseline Assessment

The initial period of observation and data collection is called the "baseline assessment." Assessing the status of symptoms before treatment informs the clinician about the extent of the client's problem and allows a rough prediction of how the problem might continue in the absence of treatment—or if the initial strategy is ineffective. The assumption we typically make is that the client's performance will look different from the baseline if the treatment is having an impact (either positive or negative). Therefore, the primary characteristic of useful baseline data is *stability* (Kazdin, 1998).

The target variable for a client with obsessive–compulsive disorder (OCD) might be the amount of time spent checking. For Viviane, a 40-year-old woman with OCD, the symptom that bothered her the most was the need to ascertain whether every appliance and electrical device had been unplugged. Although she checked the appliances at all times of the day, the problem was particularly bad before she went to bed each night, because Viviane was afraid there would be a fire while she slept. She reported spending "countless hours" every night repeatedly checking to see that her appliances were unplugged. After conducting the intake interview, the therapist continued the initial assessment by asking Viviane to collect baseline data on how many minutes she spent checking her appliances each night.

These first 7 days of Viviane's self-observations are baseline data because they were collected before the first intervention session. Note that here is an example of a case in which ample baseline data are collected without delaying treatment. In Figure 5.2, the horizontal x axis (scale from 1 to 7) represents the first week of observations. The vertical y axis (scale from 0 to 120) represents the number of minutes Viviane reported checking each evening before bed.

Stable baselines have two main features: lack of *variability* and lack of *trend*. In the first 4 days of Viviane's baseline assessment, she demonstrated remarkable variability (i.e., fluctuation) in the amount of time she spent checking before going to bed, ranging from 20 to 100

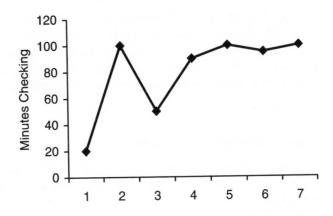

FIGURE 5.2. Viviane's baseline data: Nighttime checking during the week before treatment began.

minutes. If the therapist had begun the intervention at day 4, he would not have been confident about how much time Viviane "normally" spent checking. Was 20 or 100 minutes more representative of Viviane's behavior? After day 4, however, Viviane's checking became more stable (as illustrated by the data points being more in line with each other). The graph seems to suggest that Viviane's regular range was between 90 and 100 minutes.

Trend, the tendency to increase or decrease over time, is easy to visualize by imagining a straight line through the data, staying as close as possible to all the data points. Lack of trend is demonstrated when this line is relatively horizontal. Viviane's data are unclear on this point; there may have been an increasing trend in the amount of time that she spent checking. The therapist had only planned on a baseline assessment period of 1 week, because Viviane wanted to begin treatment right away. However, just before her first treatment session, Viviane phoned the therapist to cancel her session because a bus strike had left her without transportation. The therapist asked Viviane to continue monitoring the amount of time she spent checking in the evening, which allowed for a longer baseline assessment.

Figure 5.3 shows Viviane's checking frequency during the 7 days after her initial evaluation (represented in days 1–7, which are identical to those in Figure 5.2), as well as the unexpected additional assessment days added to the baseline (days 8–12). The clinician saw that Viviane's baseline data, including the extra days of assessment, were stable; she spent roughly 100 minutes checking each evening.

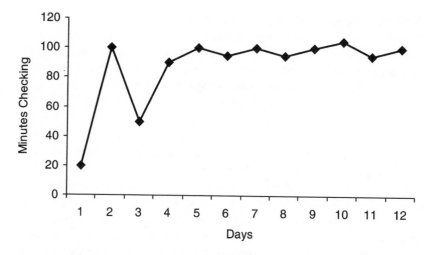

FIGURE 5.3. Baseline data for Viviane: Additional days of assessment.

Challenges to Collecting Baseline Data

It may be impractical in practice settings to collect enough observations to establish a stable baseline. Viviane's first week of data was highly variable and left open the possibility of a trend. Although Viviane subsequently collected more baseline data, in most circumstances, collecting 12 to 14 days of data would be impossible. Fortunately, one can make do with far fewer observations. In many cases, three data points are enough to provide an indication of the client's status when treatment begins.

As we discussed in Chapter 4, some clients have trouble with self-monitoring. Although motivation is usually good during the early part of treatment, compliance can be challenging during the baseline phase, because therapist and client may not yet have developed a solid working alliance. In client populations in which the clinician anticipates this problem, a once weekly measure given prior to the first treatment session is a better choice. Of course, if the therapist is attempting to collect baseline data with a measure given once per week, it would take at least 3 weeks to establish a good baseline—an obvious problem in most cases. (As we have said before, however, one data point is better than none.)

An alternative to self-monitoring between sessions is to use the client's recall. Although not ideal, the client could spend the first few minutes of the first session recollecting his or her behaviors over the past week. These retrospective data are prone to bias, but they still may help the clinician to establish some form of a baseline and are preferable to collecting no baseline data at all. If the client has difficulty recording data on a daily basis, the therapist could recommend that the client phone in (or send an e-mail) to report on the target behavior(s) one or more times between sessions. Although the reports would again rely on the client's memory, it is much easier to recall a few days observations than a whole week.

The client who comes to treatment with vaguely articulated problems poses other challenges to collecting baseline data. In this case, we tend to spend a few sessions determining the best measures for the client. In other cases, the therapist may need to intervene immediately (e.g., due to fear of client self-harm or a short time frame for therapeutic work), precluding the collection of baseline data. In challenging situations such as these, one option is to use a global standardized measure, some examples of which we discussed in Chapter 4. These measures assess a variety of problems (e.g., depression, anxiety, eating behavior) and are likely to hit on at least one problem relevant to a given client. In addition, the therapist may want to rely on the client's retrospective ratings of his or her problem behaviors once the Treatment Plan is established.

Our discussion has focused primarily on collecting *daily* baseline data to minimize the amount of time that passes before the intervention begins. Another strategy for frequently occurring problems is to gather data over an even shorter time period. Examples include an hourly record of the frequency of swearing for a child with conduct problems or of obsessional intrusions for a client (like Viviane) with OCD. In this way, a single day of recording can generate multiple data points to serve as a baseline (although we would naturally be wary of assuming that any single day is typical of a client's functioning).

Graphing Progress During Treatment

If the baseline data are relatively plentiful and stable (meaning little variability and no trend), then the therapist can more confidently project the client's future performance on the target variable in the absence of treatment (Kazdin, 1998). Given Viviane's baseline data, shown in Figure 5.4, we would project no change in her nighttime checking behavior if no treatment were provided, as indicated by the hypothetical data plotted after the solid vertical line.

Figure 5.4 shows Viviane's projected future checking without treatment, in addition to her actual progress during treatment. The solid vertical line represents the beginning of the first phase of treatment. As indicated on the graph, Viviane responded well to the first

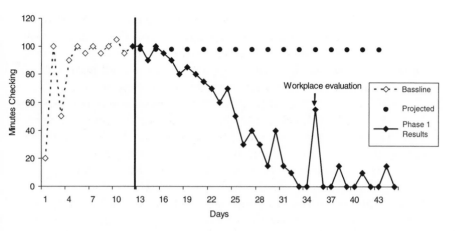

FIGURE 5.4. Baseline and Treatment Phase I for Viviane.

phase of treatment. The amount of time that she spent checking at night decreased at a relatively constant rate, although Viviane did have occasional bad days in which she saw some of her progress slip back. For instance, Viviane spent 55 minutes checking on the evening prior to her annual performance evaluation at work (as indicated by the arrow in Figure 5.4). Viviane experienced a great deal of stress prior to her evaluation, which had an impact on her checking behavior, but on the subsequent evening she did not check at all. By the end of Phase 1, the amount of time she spent checking in the evening ranged from 0 to 15 minutes. The graph helped to reinforce the fact that Viviane had made steady, yet dramatic, reductions in her nighttime checking behavior over the course of treatment. The next phase of treatment focused on some of her other OCD symptoms.

GRAPHING PROGRESS WITH MICROSOFT EXCEL

By 1996, nearly 75% of psychologists used computers in their practice, but most used them only for word processing, according to a survey by Rosen and Weil (1996). The prospect of using technology in a therapeutic context can be intimidating to those with basic-level computer skills. However, graphing client data is relatively easy and accessible. Even without a computer, graphs can be sketched out the "old-fashioned way" (with pencil and graph paper) to the same benefit. Nevertheless, using a computer spreadsheet to produce graphs is very easy, and below we provide step-by-step instructions for graphing in Microsoft Excel. Our aim has been to give instructions that are basic enough even for those who have never used a spreadsheet program. Others who are familiar with spreadsheets may find some helpful hints about organizing data relevant to treatment progress.

Although there are other spreadsheet programs that one can use (e.g., SPSS, Lotus), Excel is probably a more popular program. Some word-processing programs produce graphs but are less flexible than a spreadsheet program. Generating a new graph for a week's worth of data (5 to 7 data points) should take less than 5 minutes. Adding data points to a previously established graph takes less than a minute. Many online resources and books are available to assist with the mechanics of using Excel. We used *Using Excel 5 for Windows* (Nossiter, 1995) as a guide for this chapter. Because much of the learning with these programs comes from trial and error, simply playing around with the program may be the best way to learn the functions that best match individual style. We have summarized some of the steps involved in graphing data, beginning with the most basic:

1. First, open the Excel program by clicking on the Excel icon from your program manager or desktop, or choosing Excel from the Start menu. The data sheet window will appear; it looks like a blank table with columns labeled A, B, and so on, and numbered rows. Enter the dates that the data were collected across Row 1, as shown below:

10-Sep-02	11-Sep-02	12-Sep-02	13-Sep-02	14-Sep-02	15-Sep-02	18-Sep-02

2. Enter the assessment data in Row 2 (under the dates). In this example, the client is tracking the number of minutes he spends crying each day of the week.

10-Sep-02	11-Sep-02	12-Sep-02	13-Sep-02	14-Sep-02	15-Sep-02	18-Sep-02
75	80	65	75	55	45	50

3. To label your data (i.e., "minutes crying"), leave an empty column to the left of the data and type in the appropriate label. When you create the graph, this label will appear in the legend. More than one measure can be included on the same worksheet, even if one measure is collected weekly and the other is collected every 2 weeks (i.e., minutes crying and the BDI).

4. To graph the data, select (highlight) the labels and the data in Rows 1 and 2 (i.e., dates and minutes spent crying), and then go to the Excel toolbar and click on the "Chart Wizard" icon. A window will appear that asks if the selected data are correct. The window will present the column and row number of the first data point, then a colon followed by the column and row number of the last data point. If correct, click "Next." (If not, correct the data, then click "Next").

5. Select (click on) the chart you desire. The default is column; in our examples, we have used line charts. Click "Next."

6. Select a format for the chart. (The default is fine.) Click "Next."

7. View how the chart will look and make changes, if necessary. Click "Next."

8. Add Titles:
  a. Chart title (e.g., client name, type of behavior). For Figure 5.5, we used "Daily Crying Episodes."
  b. Category (*x*) Axis: time (e.g., dates, days of the week, session number).
  c. Value (*y*) Axis: amount (e.g., minutes spent crying, compliance, number of negative thoughts, calories consumed).

9. Chart Location: The default is to keep the graph as an object below the data on the sheet that you are already using. This option works fine; you will be able to save the graph and make additions to it later. You may also choose to place it as an object in another sheet or as a new sheet.

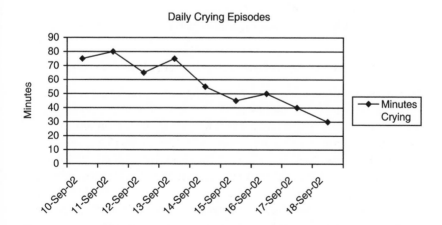

FIGURE 5.5. Example Excel graph.

10. Click "Finish." The graph is complete. If you have followed the directions listed here, using the example data provided in step 3, your graph should look like the one in Figure 5.5.

11. Adjusting chart size and placement involves a little tinkering. To move the chart, click in the chart box and hold down the mouse button while positioning. To adjust size, use the mouse pointer on the outline at the designated points (the squares on the chart outline). To adjust the style—such as line thickness, style (dotted, dashed, or solid), data points (triangles, squares, or circles)—double-click on the chart. You can now adjust patterns, font, and properties, and also point at a place on the chart and right-click with the mouse to get a menu of options.

12. Save the file by going to "File" and then "Save As" at the top of the screen.

13. At the next therapy session, ideally the client will provide more data. Add the new data by opening the saved file, typing in the new data (add dates to Row 1 and data to Row 2). To add the data to the graph you made earlier, click once on the graph. Go to "Chart" on the toolbar, and then to "Add Data." When your "Add Data" window appears, select your new data on the spreadsheet with the mouse by outlining the new data points (the outline will appear as a dashed line). The range of new data will appear automatically in the "Add Data" window. Hit "OK." You can also add the new data by clicking once on your graph. Your old data will be outlined on the spreadsheet with a heavy border. In the bottom right corner of the border, you will see a small square. Place your pointer on the small square and then drag with your mouse, so that your new data are also outlined. The new data will be added automatically to the graph.

Using "AutoFill" to Save Time Entering Treatment Dates

AutoFill saves time when you are entering dates (and other data series). This feature completes a series when you enter the first value in the series. For example, if you enter the date "10-Sep-02", then AutoFill will complete the series for you (e.g., 11-Sep-02, 12-Sep-02, 13-Sep-02 . . .). To use AutoFill, type the first number in the series into cell A1 (or any other cell). Select the cell (e.g., A1) by clicking on it once. Cell A1 will now have a heavy border around it. Notice the lower right corner of the border. The little square in the lower right corner is called the "fill handle." Using the mouse, aim at the fill handle, and the pointer turns into a black cross. Drag the fill handle through cell J1 (for example). You will see that each cell in the range is surrounded by a faint outline. Release the mouse button and the column headings will be automatically filled in, in this case beginning with 10-Sep-02 and ending with 19-Sep-02. AutoFill works with numbers, days of the week, months, and dates. All you do is type in the first value, drag, and release.

Separating Baseline Data from Intervention Data

Students or part-time clinicians will probably have no trouble remembering the point at which they began an intervention or changed treatment strategies, but busy practitioners may benefit from using simple visual cues to clarify the graphed data for each client. The most basic visual cue involves separating baseline data (in which one looks for stability) from data collected during therapy (in which one obviously hopes for signs of improvement). The same visual cue can be used to distinguish different phases of treatment. To separate baseline data from intervention data (or to separate different phases of therapy), remove the line connecting them. Click once on the data point prior to the line you want removed (Point A in Figure 5.6).

Then click once on the next data point (Point B in Figure 5.6). Both Point A and Point B will be highlighted. Go to "Format" and "Selected data point." At the window, go to "Line" and select "None." Click "OK" and the line will be removed (see Figure 5.7). (If the legend on

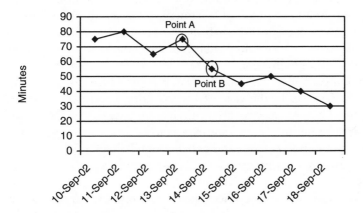

FIGURE 5.6. Separating Phases of assessment.

Daily Crying Episodes

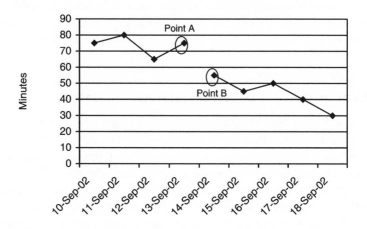

FIGURE 5.7. Illustration of baseline separated from Treatment Phase I.

the chart becomes too confusing or is unnecessary, remove it by click-ing on it and pressing the delete key.)

Inserting Arrows to Highlight Important Dates or Sessions

Another simple tool to maximize the utility of the graph is the use of arrows to point to an important date or session. Examples include the initiation of a new phase of treatment, a change in medication, or an event in the client's life, such as the breakup of a relationship. Al-though arrows are certainly useful for the clinician, they are potentially more helpful in situations in which the clinician is sharing the graph with someone else, such as the client, a supervisor, or members of a case conference. In the case of Viviane (discussed earlier; see Figure 5.4), the therapist used an arrow to demonstrate to Viviane the link be-tween the amount of stress she experienced on the evening prior to her yearly evaluation at work and her checking behavior. Viviane used this experience as a reminder that she is particularly at risk for a lapse dur-ing times of great stress.

To insert an arrow, select the "Drawing" icon from the toolbar, click on the "Arrow" icon once, and place the cursor at the point on the graph where the arrow should begin. Hold down the mouse button while drawing up to where the arrowhead should be, and then release the button.

Adding a Trendline

A trendline is a straight line running through the center of the data, staying as close as possible to each of the data points. Naturally, no collection of client data will fall on a perfectly straight line and, by definition, a trendline is calculated to have as much of the data above the line as below it. (Technically, it is departures from the line that are balanced above and below the line.) In creating a trendline, extreme changes in behavior are weighted more heavily. This means that a small lapse in progress will alter the trendline somewhat, but a large relapse will alter it quite a bit. Trendlines are especially useful in the case of erratic data, because they illustrate the slope, that is, whether the erratic data are generally increasing, decreasing, or staying the same. Trendlines are also helpful in comparing progress across different phases of treatment.

Adding a trendline to a graph is easy with Excel. After clicking once on the graph, go to "Chart," select "Add Trendline" from the menu, and click "OK." Figure 5.8 shows the earlier example with a trendline added.

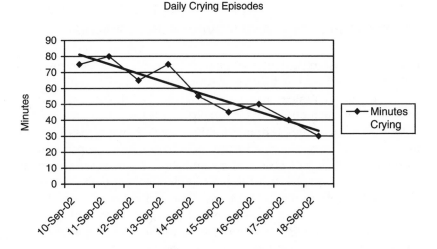

FIGURE 5.8. Illustration of trendline.

Printing the Graph

Simply pressing the printer icon in Excel will print both your graph and the raw data, if the graph is located in the worksheet with your data. If you want to have the graph fill the entire page, click once on the graph (to select it) and then go to "Print." It is a good idea to use the "Print Preview" feature before printing from Excel.

Additional Graphing Resources

Readers interested in more detailed guidance on using Excel for graphing single-subject design methodology (common for behavior-analytic research) are referred to Carr and Burkholder (1998). Additionally, for readers who would like a broader array of graphing options, *More Than a Thousand Words* by Mark Mattaini (1993) is an excellent resource. Written for social workers, this book offers sensible and creative techniques to develop and modify concepts such as time lines, single-subject designs, and family mapping, emphasizing techniques that reduce the clinician's time and effort.

For clinicians who prefer to create paper-and-pencil graphs, we have found it helpful to develop a blank template for some common scale ranges (e.g., 0–100 and 1–10). By keeping blank copies of the graphs handy, we have a ready-made grid to use when we start graphing a new domain for a client.

REVIEWING PROGRESS AND MOVING ACROSS PHASES

One of the most important aspects of graphing is reviewing progress with the client. Across theoretical orientations, direct feedback is a common clinical strategy to review progress (Goldfried, 1980). Therapists use their own observations to help clients become more aware of what they are (or are not) doing, thinking, and feeling across a variety of situations. Progress Reviews can include multiple components, including both therapist observations and more formalized assessment data. Including graphs in a Progress Review enhances the therapist–client collaboration, helps client and therapist focus on overall patterns, and directly aids in revising and creating future treatment goals. We discuss Progress Reviews more fully in the next chapter, and we consider the role of graphing in this process here.

In reviewing the graph of data that have been collected during active treatment, both the *magnitude* and the *rate* of change are important. Magnitude of change refers to changes in the mean or average level of the behavior from one assessment period to another. Rate of change refers to changes in the pattern or trend of the data and to how quickly change is occurring. Magnitude and rate of change are readily apparent on a graph.

Figure 5.9 shows BDI scores with trendlines across the baseline and two phases of treatment for a 68-year-old client called Toby. The graph demonstrates a drop in the magnitude of Toby's depression between the baseline and the end of Treatment Phase I, indicating that his level of depression declined during the first 2 months of therapy. In Phase I, Toby was receiving interpersonal psychotherapy as well as antidepressant medication. Because of the sexual side effects associated with his antidepressant, Toby abruptly stopped taking his medication approximately 6 weeks into Phase I of treatment.

When Phase II began, Toby was more depressed. Over the course of Phase II, Toby's magnitude of depression was lower than it had been at baseline but about equal to the mean depression level during Phase I. This does not convey the whole story, however, because the rate of change is important as well. Toby's depression was declining at a relatively rapid rate during the first 2 months of treatment. Although Phase II began at the point at which he experienced a return of depression, his depressive symptoms did not improve during Phase II, perhaps due in part to Toby's decision not to take medication.

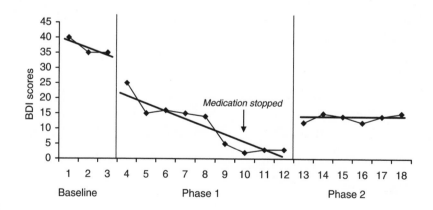

FIGURE 5.9. Magnitude and rate of change of Toby's Beck Depression Inventory scores.

CASE EXAMPLE

In Chapter 3, we introduced a 15-year-old high school sophomore named Peter, who had problems with panic as well as difficulty maintaining weight due to a fear of vomiting. We use Peter's case to illustrate how graphing can be a useful tool for giving feedback to clients.

Developing the Initial Treatment Plan

Recall from Chapter 3 that the aims in the first phase of Peter's treatment were to minimize his suicide risk and improve his depressed mood. In the second phase of treatment, the therapist and Peter chose to focus on his panic attacks and avoidance. This issue was a priority for Peter because summer school had begun, and, wary of falling behind, he wanted to be able to tolerate being in the classroom to keep up with his classes. Peter's weight loss was partially addressed in the second phase of treatment by having him meet with a nutritionist, plan three balanced meals a day, and monitor how many meals he ate each day. We begin this example with Peter's Problem List and his treatment aims, measures, and strategies for the second phase of treatment (see Figures 5.10 and 5.11).

	Client endorsed?
1. Depressed mood	√
2. Suicidal ideation	√
3. Lack of pleasant activities	
4. Inadequate nutrition and weight loss	
5. Daily panic attacks	√
6. Avoidance of places and situations where panic attacks occurred	√
7. Perfectionism and high self standards	
8. Inability to maintain close relationships	√
9. Fear of vomiting	√
10. Inability to distract from negative thoughts	√

FIGURE 5.10. Peter's Problem List.

Treatment Phase II	Date: July 3, 2002

Aims: **1.** Decrease the number of daily panic attacks

2. Decrease avoidance of feared situations (e.g., the classroom) and objects (e.g., food)

3. Maintain improvements in depressive symptoms

Measures: **1.** Monitor number of panic attacks daily
(attach graph)
2. Maintain a diary of exposure to feared situations

3. Weekly Beck Depression Inventory

4. Record number of meals consumed each day

Strategies: **1.** Relaxation training (e.g., progressive muscle relaxation, diaphragmatic breathing)

2. Thought monitoring and challenging (e.g., fear of being trapped, vomiting in public)

3. Interoceptive and situational exposures (e.g., to dizziness, nausea, public places)

Date for Phase II Progress Review: September 25, 2002

FIGURE 5.11. Peter's Treatment Plan: Phase II.

Conducting the Baseline Assessment

Recall that the goal for baseline data collection is to establish a reliable sense of the client's symptoms or functioning before treatment begins. One looks for stability in the baseline data, illustrated by a lack of variability and trend. With a stable baseline, the clinician has a clear comparison point for future assessment. When Peter and his therapist decided to move on to address his panic attacks in Phase II, Peter began keeping track of the number of panic attacks he was having each day. As he went to bed each night, Peter made a note of how many panic attacks he had experienced that day.

When Peter brought his notes on the frequency of panic attacks to his therapist, she used Excel to generate the first week of Figure 5.12, which includes Peter's data not only for the baseline but also for Treatment Phase II. During the baseline, Peter was having three to five panic attacks each day. Overall, there was little evidence of a trend (ei-

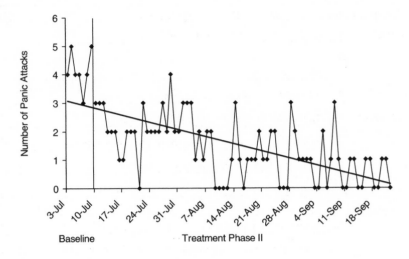

FIGURE 5.12. Frequency of panic attacks for Peter.

ther decreasing or increasing) over the week of the baseline. Note that Peter's therapist could have asked him to begin collecting this information a few weeks in advance for a longer baseline, given that she anticipated they would work on panic during Phase II. However, the therapist decided that one week's worth of baseline data was sufficient, and she began to implement her plan for Phase II intervention strategies with Peter on July 10.

Graphing and Reviewing Progress

As reflected in the Treatment Plan shown in Figure 5.11, Peter agreed to carry out four measurement tasks during Phase II of his treatment, three of which he recorded in his daily panic diary. In addition to jotting down the number of panic attacks he had each day, Peter also kept note of the challenging situations (e.g., classrooms, grocery store) he entered each day. This information was important because Peter had used avoidance to minimize the frequency of his panic attacks in the past, and a major treatment goal was to increase his mobility. From this diary, the therapist noted the number of situations Peter approached each day, as well as the number of panic attacks.

As we mentioned in Chapter 3, Peter's first phase of treatment partially addressed his eating habits. Although his nutritionist continued working with Peter to address the concerns with his eating during Phase II, his therapist wanted to monitor his eating in a basic way, because she was still concerned about his health. Accordingly, Peter agreed to tally the number of meals he ate each day. Because Peter was already making a daily rating of panic attacks and challenging situations, Peter's therapist added a column to the panic diary for Peter to record the number of meals he ate.

Finally, Peter completed the BDI each week in the waiting room before his session. Peter's measurement plan did involve a fairly large amount of self-monitoring, but his therapist judged the plan to be feasible given his high level of motivation for treatment and that just one piece of paper was required for all of the self-monitoring. For the average client, monitoring one behavior at a time may be more realistic.

When Phase II of treatment began, the therapist and Peter were focusing primarily on reducing the number of panic attacks he was experiencing each day. In session, Peter learned how to control his breathing and to relax his body. He began to practice progressive muscle relaxation twice a week (between sessions) and diaphragmatic breathing daily. Peter began to incorporate cognitive strategies into his day-to-day life (e.g., challenging catastrophic interpretations of his bodily symptoms). The frequency of Peter's panic attacks began to decline (see Figure 5.12). In the third week of treatment, Peter began practicing exposure to the sensations of anxiety (i.e., interoceptive exposure) by hyperventilating, spinning in a chair, and breathing through a straw. Peter experienced a slight increase in the frequency of his panic attacks during this time, having between two and four panic attacks a day. In reviewing his graph, Peter attributed this increase in the frequency of panic attacks to the shift in therapeutic strategies (now involving interoceptive exposure).

Although the review of Phase II was not scheduled until the end of September, Peter's therapist began generating graphs of Peter's daily panic attacks, beginning in the fifth week of Phase II. Peter and his therapist looked at a graph of his panic attacks approximately once every 2 weeks thereafter, although the frequency of sharing the graphs would be a matter of personal therapist style. Because the therapist entered the data into Excel every week, it took about 2 minutes to produce a graph of Peter's progress.

Peter also chronicled his daily exposures to feared situations and the number of meals he was eating daily. Even before exposure to feared situations was explicitly part of the therapeutic intervention, Peter began reporting occasional visits to his school or to a trusted friend's house. As treatment progressed, the number of activities Peter engaged in each day increased, from a range of 0–2 in the first 3 weeks, to a range of 1–4 in the following weeks. Peter met and even exceeded the goals he set for himself each week, and the therapy progressed at a steady pace. By the sixth week of the intervention, Peter was no longer fearful of leaving his home and was increasingly able to enter situations he had avoided for more than a year. Although Peter was keeping track of his meals and the number of challenging situations he entered each day, the therapist chose not to generate regular graphs, as she did with the number of panic attacks. This turned out to be an unfortunate oversight.

Peter's eating did not increase or stabilize over the course of the second phase of treatment. In the first 2 weeks of Phase II (immediately following an intervention by the nutritionist on July 7), Peter reached his aim of eating three meals a day at least 50% of the days in each week. Over time, however, Peter began to have greater difficulty fulfilling this aim. Both the therapist and Peter were focused primarily on decreasing the frequency of panic attacks and minimizing his avoidance of feared situations, so Peter's increasing avoidance of food (and diminishing appetite) remained largely overlooked until the Progress Review at the end of September.

As with many multiproblem clients, it can be challenging to attend to all of the relevant issues. In Peter's case, avoidance of food was included among the treatment aims of Phase II, but the strategies used to address his eating were secondary to the attention paid to panic and avoidance. In retrospect, Peter's therapist wished she had printed graphs of his meals and avoidance as often as graphs of Peter's panic attacks were generated. Even though Peter had been collecting these data, the therapist did not notice the trend without graphing them. In preparation for the Progress Review of Phase II of treatment, she finally did graph the data, which proved very useful for the Progress Review and contributed directly to the plan for Phase III of treatment. Figure 5.13 includes data from Peter's daily exposure to previously avoided situations, as well as his frequency of meals each day. The graph is fairly complicated, but it is illustrative of both problems (and their trendlines) on the same graph.

The final measure that Peter completed regularly was the BDI. As depicted in Figure 5.14, the therapist included the BDI scores from the first phase of treatment in the graph (higher scores indicate stronger depressive symptoms). Peter filled out the BDI once a week. The therapist was particularly concerned with Peter's depression given his sui-

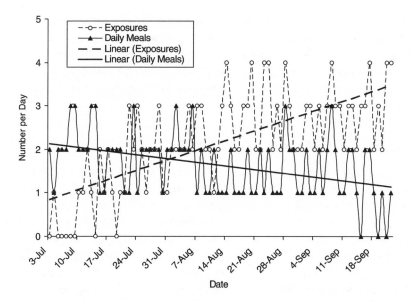

FIGURE 5.13. Peter: Exposure to feared situations and frequency of meals.

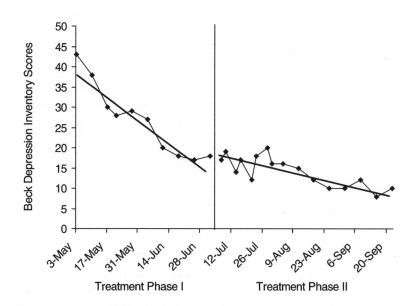

FIGURE 5.14. Course of Peter's depression across Phase I and Phase II of treatment.

cide attempt immediately prior to entering treatment. Consequently, she generated graphs of Peter's BDI scores once a month and also looked at many of the individual items on this measure. Peter showed excellent progress in reducing his depressive symptoms, for they continued to decrease even after the transition from Phase I to Phase II of treatment.

Moving across Phases

When the therapist conducted the Phase II Progress Review with Peter, she printed out all of the graphs (as shown in Figures 5.12 through 5.14) and discussed them during the session with Peter. Peter and his therapist were pleased to see the decrease both in the frequency of his panic attacks and in his depressive symptoms. They were both satisfied with the frequency of Peter's engagement in situations he had formerly avoided (i.e., exposures in Figure 5.13), but Peter's increasing tendency to avoid meals was an obvious concern. The Progress Review indicated that it was time to shift to Phase III, where they would focus primarily on his fear of vomiting, meal planning, and concerns about weight stabilization. The therapist also planned to have Peter continue monitoring his depressive symptoms and panic attacks during the third phase to watch for signs of a lapse.

RESEARCH IMPLICATIONS

Most clinicians who use our strategies will not be interested in conducting research. The PACC model does not necessitate any systematic comparison or aggregation of data across clients, and we encourage researchers and nonresearchers alike to try the approach. For practitioners interested in conducting research as a part of routine practice, we briefly address some of the relevant issues.

Single-Case Designs

Single-case designs have clear advantages for those who are interested in the development of an individual's behavior over time. Morgan and Morgan (2001) argue that single-case designs are flexible enough to be useful for practitioners and help to address the growing emphasis on demonstrating the usefulness of clinical interventions in a managed care environment. The PACC model provides a structure for the first steps toward single-case design research, which allows strong inferences about the effects of the intervention using the client as his or her own comparison condition (Kazdin, 1998).

Kazdin (1998) described the basic considerations for conducting single-case design research. The first requirement is ongoing assessment, which is obviously a main tenet of the PACC model as well. Second, separate phases of treatment (e.g., baseline, treatment, alternative treatment) are necessary for conducting single-case design research. This consideration is also quite compatible with the phase-based PACC model. Finally, there are limitations in the type of questions appropriate for single-case design research; that is, the therapist can address questions related to how well various strategies work with a particular client. The design is not equipped, however, to examine interactions of client and therapist factors in relation to treatment, because there is no way to assess and control for all of the relevant factors in the therapeutic relationship. Although the PACC model is not designed to translate the outcome for a given client into "research findings," our model is compatible with research techniques for those practitioners who do wish to make predictions and attempt to replicate their findings across a number of clients.

SHORTCUTS FOR THE BUSY CLINICIAN

In this chapter, we have argued that graphing serves to (1) enhance therapist–client collaboration, (2) help the client and therapist focus on the bigger picture, (3) increase the client's sense of self-efficacy, and (4) help revise and create future treatment goals. Given these benefits, why do so few therapists actually graph their clients' progress? The number one barrier is likely to be a lack of concrete data to put on a graph. But for those therapists who *are* measuring change, why do they still hesitate to graph? We believe that many therapists overestimate the time involved in the process of entering and graphing data, and we hope the description and examples in this chapter provide reassurance that this assumption is simply not true. Although first-time users of programs such as Excel may feel intimidated at first, only a little practice is required to feel comfortable with the basics. Once therapists get a handle on how to create graphs, 5 minutes (or less) are required to enter the client's data on a weekly basis. Most clinicians find graphs to be a visual reward for all of the effort that has been put into the measurement process. Whether the data suggest improvement, relapse, or something in between, graphing is a concrete and meaningful way to help the client get the most out of treatment.

CHAPTER 6

REVIEW OF PROGRESS

With graphs in hand, the clinician can take advantage of the data collected throughout therapy to determine how the client has fared with the chosen treatment approach. The Progress Review is an opportunity for therapist and client to look at how therapy is going, with an eye toward potentially modifying the treatment plan, moving to a new phase of treatment, or ending therapy. We also review strategies for managing client resistance and boosting motivation, as well as intervening in those cases when the Progress Review suggests that the change process has stalled.

Simply measuring a client's problems will not by itself improve the quality of treatment; it is necessary to take time to review the measures formally in the context of the overall treatment plan. Measuring change in a relatively continuous way allows the clinician flexibility and confidence in treatment planning. Regular reviews of progress do require a time commitment, but the objective of the review is to promote better quality treatment. We find that treatment is more efficient when we review progress on a regular basis, because it allows us to recognize problems and successes rapidly, which is especially important for cases in which we must work within short time constraints.

In some respects, the Progress Review serves as a follow-up to the original therapeutic contract. Much has been written about the value of negotiating a therapeutic contract. In the PACC approach, each phase of the Treatment Plan serves as an elaborated version of a therapeutic contract, and the Progress Review determines whether the contracted plan is evolving as expected. Explicitly establishing and appraising treatment aims enhances the therapeutic alliance, engages the client as an active participant in the therapy process, and links specific treatment interventions to concrete aims (Gottman & Leiblum, 1974). The PACC Progress Review also promotes open discussion between client and clinician regarding the goals and tasks of treatment.

When the Treatment Plan includes a well-researched treatment intervention, it may be tempting to assume a Progress Review is unnecessary, because the treatment has already been "validated." However, empirical support for the treatment approach is distinct from an individual client's progress. Even the best-researched treatments are not perfectly effective for every client. The only way to determine whether a particular client is improving is to evaluate progress directly. We now consider some of the practical issues involved in conducting this individualized review.

STRATEGIES FOR IMPLEMENTING A PROGRESS REVIEW

The Progress Review is based on a particular phase of the Treatment Plan. The focus of the review is not so much on whether the aims have been met as on the degree of progress the client has made. Some clients show much faster progress than expected, whereas others may even deteriorate during a given phase of treatment. Still others show gains only on a subset of the aims for a given phase. Each possible outcome of the Progress Review is useful information for deciding how to direct the next phase of treatment.

You Cannot Fail a Progress Review

Evaluating treatment progress can become threatening for both client and therapist if they perceive the process as a report card, with a judgment of "pass" or "fail." Although some organizations may frame outcome monitoring in this way, a more constructive approach is to see the process as an ongoing effort to improve quality through setting goals, measuring progress, and reevaluating the goals. Even the most seasoned and gifted therapists reformulate treatment aims as they see that some strategies work more or less effectively than anticipated. The goal of the Progress Review is not to anoint or criticize the therapist, but to provide the information necessary to guide the Treatment Plan, so that time is not wasted on an intervention strategy that is not working.

For example, Abigail was a 13-year-old girl whose parents brought her to counseling because her grades had plummeted after the transition to high school. Abigail's parents also felt she was spending too much time alone in her room, surfing the Internet. In her evaluation, the school counselor agreed that Abigail was socially isolated, and she also identified a mild learning disability. This issue was the main focus of Phase I strategies, including weekly tutoring, extra time for in-class quizzes, and anxiety management skills (e.g., breathing and relaxation strategies). At the Progress Review 2 months into treatment, the counselor found that Abigail was doing better in the classroom (e.g., participating more), but her grades and social isolation had not improved.

During the progress review, the counselor asked Abigail to talk a bit more about her view of why she had such difficulty making new friends and raising her grades. Abigail disclosed that her parents were fighting all the time, which made it difficult for her to concentrate on studying. Also, Abigail was ashamed of their fighting, which made her reluctant to invite friends over. The school counselor reconceptualized the case after the Progress Review, referring Abigail and her parents to family therapy and changing her own strategies to focus more on getting Abigail involved in after-school activities and study halls.

Routine clinical practice relies heavily on trial and error. No single approach can solve every problem that clients bring to treatment. The therapist's responsibility is not to get it right the first time, but to keep trying new strategies and to check the success of each new phase of treatment in terms of bringing the client closer to his or her overall treatment goals. In this light, even a Progress Review that reveals no movement toward the aims of treatment is worth doing, because it clarifies the situation and provides an opportunity to change the treatment plan.

Establish a Date for the Review in Advance

When we discussed the elements of the Treatment Plan in Chapter 3, we mentioned setting a date for the Progress Review in advance. On what basis does the clinician set this date? Conceptual issues (e.g., how soon change is expected) and practical issues (e.g., the timing of vacations) are important factors. We have used a general guideline of setting Progress Review dates at least every 3 months, and in many cases we use a shorter time line. This guideline has been practical in our use of the PACC method in a range of outpatient treatment settings with diverse client problems. Three months usually permits some progress even on challenging treatment aims, but it is not so long that an ineffective strategy will have been used for an excessive amount of time. We consider 3 months to be a *flexible* guideline for the outside boundary of when the Progress Review should be scheduled. A Progress Review should be conducted anytime there is reason to be concerned about the effectiveness or appropriateness of the Treatment Plan. Alternatively, some therapists may prefer to conduct a Progress Review following a certain number of sessions. This kind of schedule may be especially appropriate for intensive treatments that require multiple sessions each week, in settings where clients are in treatment for a limited amount of time, or during a maintenance or relapse prevention phase when sessions occur infrequently (e.g., monthly booster sessions).

Clinicians may be tempted to postpone an established review date if a client has missed several sessions, or if a significant life event has required crisis intervention. In fact, these are exactly the kinds of situations in which a Progress Review can be helpful. When a client's attendance is erratic or compliance has been low, the therapist may feel the intervention has not had a fair shot because it was not fully implemented. Rather than putting off a review because of this problem, we advocate thinking of poor attendance or compliance as valuable data for treatment planning. If a client is frequently missing sessions, the therapist may plan a phase of treatment that addresses whatever issue is interfering with attendance—whether that is motivation, readiness to change, or some aspect of the client's life circumstances. These interventions to get the treatment back on track can be very brief, and the Progress Review can help to determine whether they are needed.

Consider the Treatment Setting

The PACC approach is flexible enough to apply in most treatment settings. The Progress Review may need to be adapted for those practitioners who work with more transient populations, who do short-term treatment, or who have particular reimbursement constraints. For example, in some treatment settings, government-sponsored insurance requires a treatment review every 30 days. Although the aims will be more modest than for a longer treatment period, the process and benefits of conducting the review are the same.

It may be difficult to set realistic goals for change in very short-term care. In some settings (e.g., day treatment or partial hospital programs), clients have multiple, serious, and long-standing problems, yet their insurance covers only 2 weeks of intensive treatment. In such settings, treatment aims often focus on connecting the client to longer term services (e.g., outpatient care) and stabilizing medications. The Problem List and the aims of the brief treatment phase may be wildly mismatched, because the aims have to be realistic for the time frame. It is perfectly acceptable to monitor progress on aims such as establishing transfer of care or socializing a client to therapy. These short-term aims prepare the client for a subsequent phase of treatment in another setting, with the opportunity to work on the more serious problems.

For example, Luna, a 48-year-old, married woman with four children, carried several psychiatric diagnoses, including posttraumatic stress disorder, major depression, and binge-eating disorder. Hospitalized for suicidal ideation and self-injurious behavior, Luna began working with a therapist in a day hospital program after discharge from the inpatient ward. Luna's insurance covered 3 weeks of treatment, and it was up to her psychiatric nurse to work with Luna to set realistic goals for the program. Using the PACC approach, the nurse developed a lengthy Problem List, including items such as hopelessness about the future, suicidal ideation, difficulty sleeping, binge eating, parenting problems, marital difficulties, lack of supports (including an outpatient therapist), flashbacks to childhood abuse, anger outbursts, self-injurious cutting, and feelings of emptiness.

Because of the short length of stay in the program, the nurse worked collaboratively with Luna to set three short-term aims: (1) to reduce the severity of depressive symptoms (as indicated by a Beck Depression Inventory score lower than 20), (2) to decrease the frequency of cutting behavior (to no more than one time each week), (3) to establish aftercare plans (including an individual therapist, outpatient group therapy, and a psychopharmacologist). Over the course of six individual sessions, Luna's nurse taught her a number of strategies intended to combat the depressed mood and cutting behavior, and they established aftercare plans.

When it came time for the Progress Review on Luna's last day in the program, Luna was very encouraged by her progress. Luna's Beck Depression Inventory (BDI) score dropped from 36 to 17; she cut herself only once over the course of 3 weeks; she had met her new outpatient therapist, enrolled in a dialectical behavior therapy program, and was scheduled to meet her new psychopharmacologist the following week. Because the chosen aims were realistic, Luna felt a sense of satisfaction and accomplishment, which in turn mobilized her for future treatment. During the progress review, Luna commented, "For the first time in my life, I've been able to step away from my laundry list of issues and focus in. And by focusing in, I think I've really been able to learn something, in part because I didn't feel as overwhelmed by what needed to be done."

Sharing the Progress Review with Clients

The Progress Review is an opportunity for the clinician to review the overall plan for treatment and make adjustments based on data about progress the client has made. Like most other aspects of the PACC model, the Progress Review can be conducted in a fully collaborative way, or the clinician can conduct the review without explicitly involving the client. Our experience with PACC suggests that collaboration greatly facilitates the process.

For example, one man we were treating for agoraphobia did not show much improvement on the Mobility Inventory (a measure of avoidance of various situations) after the first treatment phase. During his Progress Review, however, he informed his therapist that he had made arrangements to change his delivery route (at work) to include trips across bridges he used to avoid. Although he continued to avoid other situations, such as tunnels and airplane trips, the therapy had focused primarily on bridges. If the therapist had not discussed the Progress Review explicitly with this client, she may have prematurely changed course on the basis of the largely unchanged Mobility Inventory. The Progress Review discussion made clear that not only had the client stopped avoiding bridges, but also he had made a special effort to create the need to drive over them even more.

When treatment aims have been attained, sharing the data related to progress with the client may reinforce the effectiveness of the treatment and illustrate the payoff of the client's efforts at change. Even when the client is not making much progress, the Progress Review provides an opportunity for the clinician to share ideas about the lack of progress, in an effort to reengage the client in treatment or to provide a rationale for recommending a different strategy for the next therapy phase.

Consult with Colleagues

The Progress Review need not occur in isolation. We have found it very helpful to consult with other professionals involved with the case (e.g., physicians, psychiatrists, social workers, teachers) to determine whether similar perceptions of progress are occurring across various domains of functioning. Students are in the ideal situation of having a supervisor. An option for practitioners who do not have this luxury is to organize a peer supervision group involving a monthly meeting of local practitioners who gather to discuss their most difficult cases. Sharing written treatment aims and graphic representation of measures of progress can help to communicate the details of the case during such professional consultations.

CULTURAL CONSIDERATIONS IN CONDUCTING THE PROGRESS REVIEW

We discussed the importance of selecting culturally sensitive assessments in Chapter 4. Many similar concerns arise in conducting the progress review. It can be difficult to evaluate the behaviors or feelings of people from backgrounds different than our own (Hays, 1995). In making these judgments, it is important to consider cultural norms and recognize the dangers of over- or underpathologizing. For example, Hays suggests that the Euro-American emphasis on assertiveness training may not transfer well to cultures that emphasize respect, such as Native American or Asian cultures. Thus, even if the therapist and client have agreed to focus on increasing assertiveness in treatment, the evaluation of progress on this goal needs to be placed in the context of the normative behavior of the client's cultural group.

The danger in applying any cultural recommendation too rigidly is that one can fall into the trap of stereotyping individuals by assuming that they adhere to the standards reflective of their cultural group. Ideally, one can strike a balance by considering the cultural context without making assumptions that reinforce group stereotypes (Lopez, 1997). Particularly for clients from multicultural backgrounds, the clinician needs to consider the applicability of different norms. An early assessment of degree of acculturation, as discussed in Chapter 2, may help to determine which cultural norms are appropriate for a given client (Lopez, 1997). The PACC approach provides tools for maximizing the therapist–client agreement on the goals and tasks of therapy. The Progress Review serves as another opportunity for therapists to build therapeutic alliances with their clients through direct communication about progress toward therapeutic goals and priorities for future steps in treatment.

The major types of culturally based bias that influence treatment decisions involve diagnosis and judgments of symptom severity. Like other types of decision making, clinical judgment is sometimes unwittingly influenced by the client's background. There is debate about the degree of bias in psychotherapy and disagreement about which minority groups are being judged unfairly, though there is little doubt that significant problems exist in the provision of health care. Lopez (1997) concluded that the most consistent evidence for bias was observed with clients of low intelligence or low socioeconomic status. The data were somewhat consistent for racial bias in diagnostic judgments, and relatively inconsistent for gender bias. Lopez reminds us that in addition to these biases involving oppressed groups, clinical judgment bias also can be directed toward members of nonoppressed groups, such as the underdiagnosis of alcohol abuse among white clients compared to more accurate diagnostic rates for black clients (Luepnitz, Randolph, & Gutsch, 1982).

Researchers have demonstrated that people (not just clinicians) show selective recall for information that is congruent with popular stereotypes compared to information that is contradictory (Fiske & Taylor, 1984). In considering how this common judgment error might influence clinical decision making, it is easy to see one of the major advantages for routinely collecting data related to the client's problems. Without reliable and valid data, therapists may leave a session having unintentionally made a mental note of just the information that fits their preconceived beliefs. When conducting a Progress Review based on clinical impression alone, without a record of data collected from the client, decisions are less likely to be based on all the available evidence because of the selective recall to which we are all vulnerable.

CONDUCTING PROGRESS REVIEWS WITH CLIENTS WITH PERSONALITY DISORDERS

The essence of the PACC approach is the same when treating patients with Axis II disorders as those with Axis I problems, but it is helpful to consider the impact that personality disorders can have on the process of providing feedback and evaluating progress even if a personality disorder is not the primary focus of treatment. Researchers estimate that 30–50% of outpatients have a personality disorder (Koenigsberg, Kaplan, Gilmore, & Cooper, 1985), and almost half of psychiatric inpatients have a comorbid personality disorder that affects their response to treatment (Loranger, 1990). Furthermore, the presence of Axis II problems can make it difficult for the therapist, client, and other interested parties to agree on the degree and range of progress that has been made in treatment. Self-report measures can be difficult to interpret, because it is harder to report on one's own personality processes than to report acute symptoms (Henry, 1997). Furthermore, informants, such as family members or colleagues, tend to report more personality pathology than clients (Zimmerman, 1994), making it likely that incongruent indices of progress may be found.

These challenges suggest that special care should be taken to obtain multiple sources and measures of progress for Axis II problems, to be cautious in interpreting any single measure, and to be particularly sensitive in providing feedback to clients with personality disorders. Linehan (1993) reports that clients with borderline personality disorder are often especially sensitive to negative comments, so she suggests always surrounding negative feedback with positive comments. Furthermore, she suggests limiting feedback to a few problem areas during the early stage of treatment (e.g., during the Progress Review for the first phase of therapy) even though there may be few positive changes at the beginning. Negative feedback is always challenging to present regardless of the client's presenting problems, because one walks a fine line between providing realistic information about progress and further discouraging clients who may already feel demoralized.

Along these lines, Linehan (1993) proposes that clinicians focus on specific feedback about client behaviors without presuming the client's motives. Focusing on specific behaviors reduces the likelihood that clients will discount useful feedback because the therapist assumed the wrong intent. Feedback should be offered in conjunction with concrete "coaching" instructions on how to improve the undesirable behaviors. During the feedback session, Linehan recommends actively observing the client's responses and providing nonjudgmental reflection of his or her feelings. This kind of validation includes affirming that the client's behavior makes sense within his or her current mind-set. Clients vary in their potential for improvement in treatment, but when working with long-standing problems such as personality disorders, we typically target only a small amount of change for the initial phase of treatment, to maximize the likelihood that the first Progress Review will be encouraging.

The case of Andrew illustrates how an Axis II condition has an impact on both the process and outcome of a progress review. Andrew, a 44-year-old recovering alcoholic who presented with a focal problem of ambivalence about remaining in a romantic relationship, also exhibited mild social phobia, for which he requested group treatment. Initially, the therapist targeted his relationship ambivalence during Phase I with cognitive-behavioral interventions (e.g., challenging his thoughts and beliefs about the implications of either remaining in or leaving the relationship). At the Phase I Progress Review, Andrew's ambivalence ratings (which he tracked weekly) had not changed significantly, but his social phobia concerns had increased, and he expressed a strong desire to enter group treatment for social phobia. Thus, Phase II consisted of treatment of his social anxiety, with marked positive changes on several measures.

During the group therapy, Andrew's ambivalence about his relationship had been targeted as it related to his social anxiety. For example, he suspected that his fear and anxiety about the prospect of dating led him to remain in a less than optimal romantic relationship. Nevertheless, he remained deeply ambivalent about the relationship at the end of Phase II. At this juncture, Andrew's therapist conducted a full assessment of his personality and found that he met diagnostic criteria for dependent personality disorder. Obviously, this new information led her to reformulate her view of Andrew's case prior to Phase III treatment planning. She was not surprised when Andrew stated that he expected her to "provide specific advice on what [he] should do about the relationship" during the Progress Review. The therapist explored with Andrew the idea that seeking and giving this kind of advice was part of a dependent pattern of relating to others that had characterized his life for many years. This led to agreement about pursuing a longer term interpersonal treatment for dependent personality disorder. Because change occurred more slowly in this phase, assessments occurred once every 6 weeks and the phase itself lasted 8 months.

READINESS TO CHANGE AND THE PROGRESS REVIEW

As we all know, changing long-standing behaviors is not easy; repeated efforts are sometimes required. In a study of New Year's resolutions to change an unwanted behavior, Norcross and Vangarelli (1988) found that many people reported five or more years of consecutively making the same pledge before they were able to maintain their behavioral change goal for at least 6 months. Furthermore, failing to maintain change on the first attempt does not mean that later attempts will be futile. Most people who relapse will try again, often with renewed motivation. In fact, 85% of smokers who revert after an attempt to quit subsequently try again, with an advanced readiness to change (Prochaska & DiClemente, 1984).

Research on the change process indicates that individuals who relapse do not simply "spin their wheels," returning each time to baseline functioning (DiClemente et al., 1991). Clients, like everyone else, appear to learn from their mistakes, so that future efforts often represent a more effective and informed attempt. The Progress Review in the PACC approach can be used to increase the potential for learning when expected levels of change have not been achieved. By making the change process explicit and creating opportunities to discuss hypothesized barriers and facilitators of change, therapist and client increase the likelihood that a more effective change strategy can be implemented in a subsequent treatment phase.

We know that progress in therapy is related to the client's pretreatment readiness to change (Prochaska & DiClemente, 1992; Prochaska et al., 1992), and that positive outcomes are most likely when treatment strategies match the client's stage or readiness to change (Prochaska et al., 1992). Although we recommend assessing readiness to change at the initial evaluation, the Progress Review provides another opportunity to question the client's stage of change, particularly if the expected change has not been accomplished. In addition, finding that progress has not occurred in the first treatment phase does not necessarily mean that the strategies are ineffective for the client, or that the client cannot succeed in affecting long-term change. The degree of readiness to change is one reason why it may be necessary to shift strategies in a new phase of therapy. We now consider some of the other reasons for changing treatment phases.

REASONS TO MOVE TO A NEW TREATMENT PHASE

Aims Have Been Met

Everyone hopes that the Progress Review will reveal that the client has successfully achieved change toward the aims for that treatment phase and is now ready to tackle new problems in a subsequent phase. When this happy circumstance occurs, the question that remains is how much change should be evident (and how long should it be maintained) before concluding that the problem no longer needs to be a focus of treatment? Similarly, how much evidence is required to trust the pervasiveness of the change? Behavior change in the workplace will be sufficient for some clients, for example, but others may also need to change their ways of relating with family and friends. A related question concerns the reliability of different measures of change. Is an aim considered to be successfully accomplished if the client reports change and the therapist's perception is similar but the client's spouse or teacher offers a conflicting impression?

Assuming that the therapist and client feel satisfied that the central aims for the phase have been met, the next step is to return to the Problem List and determine the next focus of treatment. Obviously, we first assess whether new problems have arisen and whether the initial problems are still prioritized in the same way. Sometimes change during one phase of treatment carries over to other problems, minimizing the need to intervene directly for those issues. As therapist and client set the aims and select the measures for a new treatment phase, it will be important that the client maintain the behavioral changes already achieved. Monitoring problems from the previous treatment phase is one way to help maintain change. Alternatively, a relapse prevention program may be an essential element of the subsequent phase for some clients.

New Problems Emerge

Clients' lives do not go on hold when they enter therapy, so it is not unusual for a client to have a crisis occur while in treatment. In some cases, the crisis may be related to the primary problem, such as when a client makes a suicidal gesture. At other times, the problem will be unrelated to the treatment focus but still serious enough to warrant immediate attention. Examples might include serious illness or death of a loved one, loss of a job, or even positive events, such as a planned pregnancy. The flexibility inherent in the PACC approach allows the therapist to continue to use the system while responding to crises or major life events. At times, a stressful event may spark a change in the focus of the treatment. The therapist and client must then determine whether the situation necessitates immediate intervention or interferes with effective treatment of the original problem.

If the emerging crisis requires postponement of the original Treatment Plan, then the change in therapeutic attention effectively entails shifting to a new phase of treatment. Consequently, it will be important to consider the appropriate aims, measures, and strategies for the new phase (e.g., focusing on the stressful event), just as for any other planned intervention. An important issue is the extent to which aims and measures for the original problem may be incorporated into the new phase in the form of maintenance work or ongoing monitoring. For example, when a spouse separates from a client with anger control problems, it may be immediately necessary to address how the client will handle the separation and cope with new life changes. Nonetheless, the clinician ideally will want to continue reinforcing the anger management strategies, so the client can use already-acquired skills to respond adaptively to the estranged spouse and changed life circumstances. The challenge is to shift the treatment focus to address the new problem, so that gains made on the initial treatment focus are not completely lost.

Secondary Problems Become More Acute

The emergence of a new problem and reprioritizing an old problem are similar with respect to maintaining a balance of focus on both old and new problems. The central difference lies in the unexpected nature of a new crisis versus monitoring warning signs for long-standing problems. Old problems may become more acute (and require immediate attention) when the client has several distinct problems, such as depression and an anxiety disorder. The challenge during the initial evaluation is to determine which problem is primary or most needs direct intervention. Where possible, we try to monitor changes in the secondary problem while directly treating the primary condition. Doing so helps us feel that we will be able to recognize a worsening situation before it escalates unnecessarily. For instance, if a client were to complete a regular measure of depression, such as the BDI, while working on his body dysmorphic disorder, the therapist could identify increasing depressive symptoms and help prevent the onset of a full depressive episode.

It is often difficult to monitor multiple problems simultaneously and even more challenging to recognize in advance which problems have the potential to escalate. However, in those ideal circumstances in which there is a clear marker to indicate the worsening of a secondary problem, it can be very helpful to set a threshold at which the problem will be considered severe enough to require a shift in treatment. An obvious example is the case in which a client is being monitored for suicidal ideation; the clinician may decide that an active suicide plan demands immediate attention.

In cases in which the client is secretive about the secondary problem or finds the symptoms ego-syntonic, switching treatment phases in a collaborative manner can be difficult. For example, clients with anorexia nervosa are usually loath to agree that hospitalization or a serious intervention will be required should their weight drop to a certain level. Two strategies may help make the transition to a new phase smoother when an old problem has worsened. First, establishing agreement with the client about acceptable levels of functioning on the old problems highlights problems beyond the focus of the current treatment phase. Second, issues from the original Problem List can be monitored with routine administration of a very brief measure even if they are not selected as the initial treatment focus.

SEEKING CONSULTATION TO IMPROVE TREATMENT DELIVERY

Progress Reviews that reveal no improvement or minimal change are disappointing. The challenges for the therapist and client are to maintain hope that change can occur and to identify the reason(s) for the lack of progress. One possibility to consider is that the treatment has not been fully delivered (rather than immediately assuming that the treatment approach is ineffective). Problems implementing a treatment strategy can occur for a variety of reasons, some of which include client and therapist variables, and others that are situational. In cases in which the clinician feels that he or she has difficulty applying an intervention effectively, we have found it helpful to seek consultation before abandoning the treatment. For example, it can be difficult for therapists who are new to cognitive techniques to challenge automatic thoughts effectively. Consulting with colleagues, pursuing additional training on desired skills, or using treatment-related resources (e.g., books on specific therapeutic techniques) can all help improve the integrity of treatment delivery. Evaluating taped sessions using a therapy integrity measure, such as the Cognitive Therapy Scale (Vallis, Shaw, & Dobson, 1986), can also provide useful feedback.

Client Resistance

Psychologists disagree about the best way to define resistance, but one useful definition is "those aspects of clients' functioning that seek to maintain the status quo in their psychological lives" (Newman, 1996, p. 34). Although this definition suggests that the signs of resistance lie in client functioning, therapists can play a role as well. Another view is that resistance can be interpreted as a sign that the intervention is not appropriate for the client's present stage of change. Client resistance is related to therapist style (Miller & Sovereign, 1989), and Miller and Rollnick (1991) have developed practical strategies to minimize resistance. The bottom line is that there are several strategies the therapist can try to initiate or to restore momentum in treatment. Resistant behaviors are undeniably exasperating and interfere with the therapy process, but they also serve as valuable information that a client is not aligned with the therapist's goals or strategies.

What is resistance? Researchers have identified four major categories of resistance behaviors (Chamberlain, Patterson, Reid, Kavanagh, & Forgatch, 1984; Miller & Rollnick, 1991). First, clients sometimes *argue* with the therapist in an attempt to challenge or discount the accuracy and integrity of the treatment. Second, some clients repeatedly *interrupt* the therapist in what is interpreted as defensive behavior to resist change. Third, clients engage in *denial* by being reluctant to acknowledge responsibility for problems. Finally, by not answering questions directly or not paying attention, some clients *ignore* the therapist, a resistance strategy particularly common among adolescent clients. Each of these behaviors can be included in the therapist's formal Problem List (although potentially without client endorsement) and as part of the aims for some phases of the Treatment Plan.

The challenge for therapists is to maintain a collaborative approach in the face of client resistance (Newman, 1996). Newman suggests that the initial goal should be to gain an understanding of the resistance from a functional perspective, as a way to shed light on the client's concerns about the consequences and process of change (Newman, 1994). Table 6.1 shows 10 general strategies Newman (1994) proposed to help guide clinicians who are searching for techniques to use when a disappointing Progress Review suggests that resistance is a problem.

In their 1991 book on motivational interviewing strategies, Miller and Rollnick provide direct examples of language to use and strategies to implement reflective listening with resistant clients. The common thread among practitioners writing about resistance is the emphasis on the normality of encountering resistance and the opportunities for proactive therapist responses to minimize its negative impact.

TABLE 6.1. Ten Strategies for Overcoming Client Resistance

1. Educate the client about therapy so that the treatment rationale is clear.
2. Use the Socratic method to help clients find their own answers.
3. Provide the client with choices and an active say in the direction of treatment.
4. Collaborate and compromise rather than being overly directive or overly passive.
5. Review the pros and cons of change and of maintaining the status quo.
6. Provide empathy for the client's resistance to reduce contention and promote constructive dialogue.
7. Discuss the case conceptualization with the client.
8. Speak the client's language so that the client feels heard and understood.
9. Maximize the use of client self-direction to promote the client's active role in therapy.
10. Gently persist when a client uses subtle avoidance, rather than ignoring or forcing the problem.

Note. Adapted from Newman (1994).

Poor Motivation to Change

As discussed in Chapter 3, Miller and Rollnick (1991) conceptualize motivation as a dynamic state that fluctuates across time and varying situations. In the context of a Progress Review, if anticipated changes are not occurring, we encourage the therapist to evaluate the client's motivation level to determine whether strategies to increase motivation may be helpful.

Typically, motivation has been assessed informally in treatment, based on the client's expressed desire for help or the extent to which she or he tends to agree with the therapist. Although these informal routes are revealing, they do not necessarily help the therapist predict when change will occur (Miller, 1985). To more directly assess motivation, therapists have relied either on self-reported measures of readiness to change or a decisional balance approach. Decisional balance is a method in which the clinician assists the client in evaluating the advantages and disadvantages of maintaining versus changing behavior (Appel, 1986; Janis & Mann, 1977). The idea behind this approach is that the client's motivation to change increases as the costs of maintaining the status quo outweigh the benefits. The balance is not based solely on the number of arguments but takes into account their importance to the client. Also, the process of assessing motivation is itself likely to influence the client's incentive to change, because it emphasizes (often for the first time) the relative weight of the positive and negative consequences of continuing versus changing the problem behavior.

For example, Catalin, a 24-year-old man who had sought treatment for his severe difficulties in social situations, was making little progress toward his goal of meeting new people and making friends. He never completed between-session assignments, such as starting a conversation with a coworker, although he endorsed the appropriateness and manageability of these tasks in session. Catalin's therapist began to explore decisional balance with him in an effort to boost his motivation to attempt new behaviors. This strategy illustrated the strong conflict Catalin felt about making changes. He could list no advantages for maintaining his behavior, but he was clear about the disadvantages of changing: risking rejection, potentially looking stupid or incompetent as he tried something new, calling attention to his face (which he felt was intensely ugly), and being pitied for his social awkwardness. The disadvantages of maintaining his behavior mirrored the advantages of changing; Catalin wanted to stop feeling so lonely, begin a dating relationship, make friends, and "feel normal."

Although these advantages of change represented goals Catalin yearned to meet, they were also relatively long-term projects, whereas he felt the disadvantages of change acutely whenever he contemplated engaging in new social behavior. Understanding this dilemma allowed Catalin to begin to view his anxiety and vulnerability as "investments" toward his goals, and his therapist changed her strategy in an effort to suggest between-session exercises that promoted short-term social benefits, as well as the longer term process of building relationships.

Miller and Rollnick (1991) emphasize that poor motivation is a challenge for therapeutic skills rather than an occasion to blame or to give up on the client. If the assessment of motivation suggests that commitment to the change process is low, it may be necessary to shift the treatment focus to increase motivation, as was the case with Catalin. Table 6.2 provides a list of eight strategies that Miller and Rollnick suggest for boosting motivation. The strategies form a convenient mnemonic, running alphabetically from A through H.

The resemblance between the list in Table 6.2 and Newman's strategies for managing resistance (in Table 6.1) illustrates the linkage between motivation and resistance, and the potential for these client behaviors to be influenced in treatment. Ambivalence about, or perceived inability to change can be targeted like other issues on the Problem List by developing aims, measures, and strategies to resolve them.

TABLE 6.2. Strategies to Boost Client Motivation

Give *Advice*	Identify the problem, explain the value of change, and outline specific change strategies.
Remove *Barriers*	Reduce obstacles to change.
Provide *Choices*	Acknowledge freedom of choice and personal responsibility.
Decrease *Desirability*	Make the status quo seem less appealing than change.
Practice *Empathy*	Understand the client's meaning by use of reflective listening.
Provide *Feedback*	Make the client aware of the reality of the current situation and its consequences.
Clarify *Goals*	Help the client set realistic goals.
Actively *Help*	Directly help to enable the client to change.

Note. Adapted from Miller and Rollnick (1991). Copyright 1991 by The Guilford Press. Adapted by permission.

The Client is Ready for Termination

Once the client has experienced the desired improvement in symptoms and functioning, it is time to consider termination. In preparation for the end of therapy, it may be helpful to consider a brief final phase of treatment involving relapse prevention strategies to boost the client's skills to maintain the gains of therapy. The goals in relapse prevention are to anticipate and prevent a return to dysfunctional behavior or to promote speedy recovery from a lapse or slip before it worsens into a relapse. Assessment of relapse risk may seem a superfluous exercise when the client has already resolved the problem behavior and appears ready for termination. However, many clients continue to struggle with aspects of the problem that brought them to treatment. Some problems are more likely than others to be associated with risk of relapse, with substance abuse disorders probably leading the pack, with mood disorders close behind them. Although the rates of relapse for other problems may not be as high, it is a significant problem for most areas of clinical practice.

One challenge of implementing a relapse prevention program is explaining the rationale to the client without appearing to be pessimistic. Clinicians cannot afford to give the impression that clients are not expected to maintain their treatment gains, but clients need to understand the importance of being vigilant to prevent lapses. Writing about the tough problem of substance abuse, Marlatt and Gordon (1985) suggest conveying the logic of relapse prevention to the client in the context of other preventive measures that are taken to prepare for unlikely but serious outcomes, such as fire drills. With such a strategy, clients can usually appreciate the necessity of proactively addressing vulnerable situations. This process also can help make termination a less threatening prospect, because the client feels better prepared to handle future challenges.

Once the client understands the rationale for relapse prevention and the areas of vulnerability have been assessed, the next step is to select strategies for this final treatment phase. In general, relapse prevention is designed to help the client rehearse adaptive responses to high-risk situations, such as planning how to cope with frustration or strong cravings. Marlatt and Gordon (1985) suggest a number of potential aims and strategies for a relapse prevention phase, ranging from enlisting client support systems (e.g., family, friends) to encouraging the client to learn from failure experiences, to enhancing coping skills through the use of imagery and lifestyle modification.

Other strategies for avoiding setbacks include providing the client with booster sessions following the termination of treatment or including procedures that require minimal therapist contact, such as periodic reminder letters or phone calls (Wilson, 1992). However, the utility of booster sessions has been questioned, particularly in the treatment of obesity and smoking (Lichtenstein, 1982; Wilson, 1985). Therapists can address this concern explicitly by formulating the final (reduced contact) stage of therapy as an explicit phase of treatment, complete with its own Treatment Plan, including aims, measures, and strategies. Thus, the therapist can measure whether the aims are being met during a reduced contact phase. It can also be helpful to have the client continue self-monitoring after treatment has ended. By establishing a threshold that will indicate potential deterioration, the client knows to return to treatment before a full relapse occurs.

WHEN A LAPSE HAS OCCURRED

Because lapses are relatively common, it is important to plan in advance how to respond when a client does slip. The goal is to prevent the slip from escalating into a relapse. The range of interpretations of a lapse is illustrated in part by the multiple definitions of "relapse" in

Webster's New Collegiate Dictionary (1983). Relapse is defined first as "a recurrence of symptoms of a disease after a period of improvement." Second, relapse is "the act or instance of backsliding, worsening, or subsiding." Thus, a setback can be construed either as an all-or-none return to the disease state or as a simple instance of backsliding.

The compensatory model can be useful in dealing with relapse. In this model, the therapist avoids blaming clients for the development of their problems, but she or he expects them to compensate for their difficulties by taking responsibility for changing their behavior, even when setbacks occur (Brickman et al., 1982). This philosophy was poignantly summarized by the Reverend Jesse Jackson: "You are not responsible for being down, but you are responsible for getting up" (cited in Marlatt and Gordon, 1985, p.15). In this model, a lapse is framed as a learning experience that helps prevent further decline. Maintaining behavioral changes is a trial-and-error process, as is the learning of most new skills. In Marlatt and Gordon's (1985) relapse prevention approach, errors are expected when clients' skills are newly acquired, but with practice they become less frequent.

CASE EXAMPLE

In Chapters 3 and 5, we followed the case of Peter, a 15-year-old boy with major depression, panic disorder, and a fear of vomiting. The first phase of treatment focused primarily on Peter's suicidal ideation and depressive symptoms. In Phase II, the treatment focus shifted to Peter's panic symptoms. The Phase II Progress Review took place after approximately 3 months. As you may recall from Chapter 5, the Phase II Progress Review indicated that Peter had maintained his reduction of depressive symptoms from Phase I and had demonstrated significant improvement in his panic disorder. Peter was routinely entering previously feared situations, and the frequency of his panic attacks had decreased from four to six per day before treatment to one or none per day at the Phase II Progress Review.

Peter's therapist decided to use an entire session for the Progress Review, and Peter was very pleased to see the evidence of steady reductions in his panic and depressive symptoms. Peter had also been tracking the number of meals he ate each day, as a behavioral indicator of the intensity of his fear of vomiting. As discussed in Chapter 5, Peter and his therapist, upon inspecting the graphed data, were concerned to find that Peter had been eating fewer than two meals per day over the past 2 weeks; sometimes he went a whole day without a meal. Peter reacted to this discovery with a mixture of embarrassment and distress, stating, "It looks so much worse when I look at my meals on a graph like that. . . . It's much easier to go through a day and avoid eating and not really realize what I'm doing until I fill out my food record at the end of the day. I can't believe how bad it looks when you line all the days up."

The therapist reassured Peter that the purpose of the Progress Review was to identify problem areas as well as successes, then proposed that it was time to shift to Phase III of treatment, providing the following rationale:

1. *Aims were met.* Peter's panic attacks had decreased in frequency. He had decreased his avoidance of feared situations and maintained improvement in his depressive symptoms.
2. *Old problems were reprioritized.* Peter's fear of vomiting, as indicated by his avoidance of food, had become a serious health threat. Specifically, Peter had not gained any weight since beginning treatment, and he was consuming significantly fewer calories per day than had been recommended by his nutritionist.
3. *Relapse prevention was indicated.* Peter had been successful in combating his symptoms of depression and panic, and appeared ready to identify future high-risk situations and the appropriate coping strategies.

Peter was eager to move on to the third phase of treatment, so he and his therapist collaborated to set new treatment aims, measures, and strategies.

TROUBLESHOOTING: ANTICIPATING BARRIERS TO CONDUCTING PROGRESS REVIEWS

The intent of the Progress Review is to provide therapists with a concrete tool that can be used to design ongoing treatment plans. The Progress Review should not add to therapists' paperwork. In this final section, we address common concerns about the prospect of conducting progress reviews and barriers to their implementation.

Time Required to Prepare for and Conduct Reviews

The Progress Review may appear to require excessive time and energy. However, in implementing the PACC system, we have found that if we have been measuring progress throughout treatment, the review is primarily a matter of integrating information we have already gathered. For each of us, the first review felt somewhat laborious, because it was new, but once we had established a template (for preparing graphs, filling out the treatment phase sheets, and talking to our clients), the reviews quickly became routine. Most importantly, the review is specifically designed to promote efficiency over the course of treatment by quickly detecting problems and highlighting the most effective interventions.

Discomfort about Making the Treatment Process So Explicit

Many therapists find it strange to speak so openly with the client about the treatment process and to rely so directly on data as a main resource for clinical judgment. However, the formulation of the Treatment Plan and sharing of progress with the client is intended to foster the therapeutic alliance and enhance collaboration. Therapists can choose how extensively they discuss the Progress Review with their clients. As we mentioned earlier, a number of factors guide therapist decisions, including one's therapeutic style and the client's ability to respond to disappointing feedback. Regardless of the therapist's choice on this issue, the process of articulating a Treatment Plan and evaluating progress on the plan (either openly with the client or on one's own) will lead to more focused and demonstrably powerful treatment. The emphasis on direct collaboration with the client in no way minimizes the therapist's role as the expert on treatment for the problem. It simply clarifies the client's role in the relationship, making the client the expert on his or her experience of the problem.

Concern about a "Report Card"

As we mentioned earlier, a common concern in preparing for a Progress Review is that the client (or even the therapist) will feel he or she is being judged. As Persons (1989) notes, hearing feedback about one's progress can be unnerving for a client who fears failure or rejection.

Similarly, the review can also feel threatening to a clinician who feels that a lack of progress means he or she is in some way failing. However, unlike a report card that focuses only on past performance, the review is designed to facilitate and target the therapeutic work toward future success. In fact, the process of providing feedback can serve as an impetus to motivate change.

For example, a program developed at the University of New Mexico found that problem drinkers who received structured, personalized feedback about their alcohol use showed significantly reduced consumption (Miller & Sovereign, 1989). Therapists structured feedback for clients and helped them to understand the results of the progress review, thereby increasing the likelihood that clients would experience the review as a constructive process. When providing assessment feedback, Miller and Rollnick (1991) suggest concluding the session with a summary of the review that includes (1) the problems that emerged from the assessment, (2) the client's positive and negative reactions to the findings, and (3) an opportunity for the client to add to or correct the review summary. To this list, we would add discussing the encouraging findings from the review and determining how the results can be used to guide the next phase of treatment.

CONCLUSIONS

The Progress Review is the foundation for evaluating individual clients' progress and preparing for subsequent phases of treatment. It is the therapist's opportunity to determine whether the treatment strategies actually resulted in achievement of the specified aims. Regardless of the outcome of the review, the therapist obtains valuable information to help plan the next phase of treatment. Combining the strategies recommended in this chapter with the practical steps outlined for conducting reviews can make assessing progress easy and rewarding. Most therapy is an iterative process that involves trying various interventions, so transitioning to a new treatment phase is an expected part of being a conscientious practitioner. Shifting treatment phases can occur for a variety of reasons; some signify progress, such as resolving a problem behavior, and others follow from a mixed review, such as realizing the need to address client resistance. In either case, the information gathered from the Progress Review can help guide treatment planning. By regularly reviewing the client's progress, the therapist has the necessary data to make informed decisions in response to the wide array of treatment outcomes.

SHORTCUTS FOR THE BUSY CLINICIAN

Breaking down the Progress Review into small steps can make the process more manageable. The following list is 10 steps we use in our own Progress Reviews with clients using the PACC method:

1. Develop a convenient tracking system to anticipate upcoming progress reviews (e.g., notes in a daybook, a computer log, overleaf in the front of the client's chart).

2. If you intend to discuss the review with your client, provide him or her with notice that the review date is approaching. In the session before the review, we often ask clients to think in the coming week about their degree of satisfaction with the progress they have made and to formulate a sense of their goals and priorities for the next phase of treatment.

3. In addition, think about your own objectives for the review (e.g., celebrate progress with the client, motivate an ambivalent client) and prepare how to frame the review in the most helpful terms.

4. In preparing for the review, transform the data you have collected into a form that is easily interpreted and communicated, usually a graph (see Chapter 5 on preparing your data for visual inspection).

5. Decide whether you need to consult with other professionals or significant others, and secure written consent to do so.

6. Formulate a tentative plan for the next phase of treatment based on your interpretation of the data. Depending on the degree of collaboration in the review process, you may wait to share your ideas with the client until you hear his or her impressions of the progress thus far. Alternatively, if the client has difficulty formulating realistic goals or needs a more directive approach, then present the next phase as a more complete plan.

7. Determine how much session time you want to allot to the review process. Some therapists prefer to spend only a few minutes at the beginning of the session showing graphs to their client. Other therapists regard the review as a treatment intervention in its own right and hence use more time to discuss the data and subsequently establish a plan for the next phase of treatment.

8. Conduct the review! Share your data and impressions with the client and determine whether the client's impressions are congruent with your own. You may want to discuss discrepancies and use this information to refine the plan for the next phase of treatment.

9. If you have chosen to give feedback to other people related to the case, discuss with the client how this will occur and make a plan of action. For example, will the client discuss the results with her husband? Will you call a teacher? Does an insurer need to see a copy of a progress graph?

10. If you have concerns about the progress of the case, consult with other professionals, then complete the Treatment Plan form related to the new phase of treatment.

CHAPTER 7

ITERATIVE TREATMENT PLANNING AND ITS APPLICATIONS

This final chapter is a summary and quick reference for the PACC approach. As part of the overall review, we present a flowchart to guide decision making related to treatment planning and describe at some length a case that illustrates the application of the PACC approach to a client with multiple problems, tracing his care from intake to termination. We also discuss some of the ethical issues that may arise while using the PACC approach in practice. Finally, we offer several suggestions for how the PACC approach might be useful in various practice, research, and educational settings.

THE DECISION TREE

We constructed the Decision Tree as a flowchart to illustrate some of the choice points in treatment planning. The various boxes and arrows reflect the notion of treatment as an iterative process involving continual reflection on which strategies are (and which are not) effective for a particular client. Seasoned practitioners implicitly use such an iterative process, and other writers have also used the flowchart scheme to describe decision making in treatment planning (e.g., Gottman & Leiblum, 1974). In spite of the familiarity of the general concept, the

Decision Tree highlights some choice points particular to evidence-based treatment planning such as the PACC system (e.g., a focus on measurement). The left side of Figure 7.1 (below) shows the Decision Tree, and the right side (on page 173) provides a list of suggested questions to guide treatment planning at various stages of the treatment process. Consider these questions as a starting point, not an exhaustive index, of the issues involved in treatment planning.

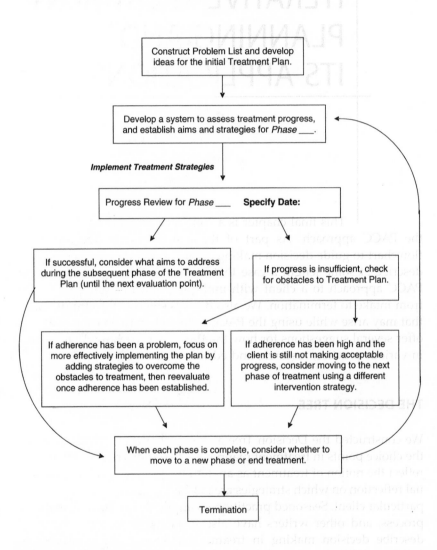

Construct Problem List and develop ideas for the initial Treatment Plan.

Develop a system to assess treatment progress, and establish aims and strategies for *Phase* ___.

Implement Treatment Strategies

Progress Review for *Phase* ___   **Specify Date:**

If successful, consider what aims to address during the subsequent phase of the Treatment Plan (until the next evaluation point).

If progress is insufficient, check for obstacles to Treatment Plan.

If adherence has been a problem, focus on more effectively implementing the plan by adding strategies to overcome the obstacles to treatment, then reevaluate once adherence has been established.

If adherence has been high and the client is still not making acceptable progress, consider moving to the next phase of treatment using a different intervention strategy.

When each phase is complete, consider whether to move to a new phase or end treatment.

Termination

FIGURE 7.1. Decision Tree.

Questions to Ask Along the Way

Problem List

- Which problems are most pressing, and what changes is the client prepared to attempt?
- Based on the time available, what problems can I realistically address?
- Based on what criteria will I choose my first line of treatment? Have I balanced the research literature with my individual client's (or group's) particular needs?

Treatment Plan

- Have I incorporated ongoing, regular assessment into my Treatment Plan?
- Am I measuring both global and individual, problem-specific concerns?
- Are my measures sensitive enough to show ongoing changes?
- Have I chosen an appropriate frequency to assess each measure?
- What criteria will I use to evaluate whether I need to alter the Treatment Plan?
- Do I have a supervisor or colleague who could offer advice on modifying my Treatment Plan?

Obstacles to Implementing Treatment Successfully

- Therapist factors: How am I going to maximize the quality of my delivery of the Treatment Plan? Have I given the initial plan a fair shot?
- Client factors: What might be interfering with my client's readiness for change (e.g., ambivalence, skills deficit, environmental contingency, problems in the therapeutic alliance)?
- External factors: How might other interested parties or circumstances be interfering with the success of treatment? Are pharmacological or other treatments at odds with my intervention?

Progress Review

- In choosing my second line of treatment, am I taking into account the scientific evidence as well as my client's particular needs and previous treatment history?
- If progress has been successful but the client still has serious problems, consider whether new aims need to be established for the next phase of the Treatment Plan.
- If repeated treatment approaches are not showing any progress, at what point will I consider a referral to another therapist or termination of treatment?
- If it is time to terminate treatment, should I first include a brief relapse prevention phase?

FIGURE 7.1. *(continued)*

The top of the Decision Tree (in the first box) illustrates the initial step of constructing the Problem List and developing ideas for the initial phase of treatment. The right top panel includes questions that are particularly relevant at this stage of treatment planning, when prioritizing problems and selecting strategies for the first phase of treatment. The second box on the Decision Tree represents the activities involved in completing the Treatment Plan for the first and subsequent phases of treatment. As we discussed in Chapter 3, the elements of the Treatment Plan include establishing aims for that phase of treatment, developing a plan for assessing progress toward those aims, and outlining basic interventions. The right panel lists important questions related to measurement and strategy selection during the development of the Treatment Plan.

As the Decision Tree reflects, the next step is to implement the planned therapeutic strategies. The date (or session number) for the Progress Review should be planned in advance. During the Progress Review, the clinician and client may feel satisfied with progress on the specified aims (see the left box below the "Progress Review" box on the Decision Tree), so treatment may either proceed to another phase to address additional aims or end. If progress has been unsatisfactory during a given phase of treatment (see the right box below "Progress Review"), then the Decision Tree provides suggestions for overcoming potential obstacles to successful treatment. If adherence has been a problem (either therapist adherence to the planned interventions or client adherence to the recommended behavior changes), then refocusing treatment to address these problems may be a viable next phase of therapy.

On the other hand, strategies that are implemented well by the therapist and faithfully attempted by the client may still fail to produce changes. In that case, the Decision Tree guides clinicians to consider moving to another phase of treatment with different strategies. This new phase may involve a different treatment strategy (e.g., shifting from cognitive therapy to interpersonal therapy for depression). Alternatively, the case may be reconceptualized, based on experiences from the first phase, and focus on altogether different aims, measures, and strategies for the new phase. The questions in the right panel of the Decision Tree provide suggestions for assessing some common obstacles to successful treatment implementation.

The bottom of the Decision Tree is related to the Progress Review. As each treatment phase is completed, clinicians naturally decide whether to proceed to a new phase of treatment or to end therapy. This decision is based partly on the client's remaining problems and partly on financial and other logistical considerations. The questions at the bottom of the right panel of Figure 7.1 are related to the choice points during the Progress Review.

In our own use of the Decision Tree, we usually have to work through several phases before termination. The goal is not to work through the flowchart as quickly as possible but to use it as a guide to many of the relevant questions raised at each decision point in treatment planning. In thinking through these questions during various stages of treatment, therapists may decide to revise the Problem List or Treatment Plan based on new information and experiences during treatment.

CASE STUDY: USING THE DECISION TREE

In the next few pages, we use the case of Xavier to illustrate movement through several phases of treatment for his various problems. Xavier's case, which is typical of some treatment settings in which clients are often seen for multiple episodes of care, would be atypical in other settings in which short-term care or crisis management is the norm. Xavier initially sought psychotherapy because he recognized that his anger was getting the best of him and causing problems in his family. He was also depressed and had a hard time coping with the demands of family and work, as well as financial difficulties. As we describe below, after the first two phases of treatment, Xavier left therapy. He subsequently returned to the clinic on two occasions: the first to address his increasingly unhappy marriage, and later to grapple with religion and spirituality.

Xavier's therapist used measurement to determine when each phase was sufficiently complete to move on to another. In this case example, different phases of treatment involved therapeutic approaches from different theoretical orientations, and multiple treatment providers were involved at times. The case illustrates the iterative process of the PACC model and use of the Decision Tree as Xavier's initial goals for psychotherapy were met and other concerns arose.

Phase I

Problem List and Initial Treatment Plan

Xavier, a 30-year-old electrician, initially sought therapy to address his "problems with anger and depression." He described a destructive pattern of episodes in which his anger would suddenly escalate and he would yell at his children and his wife. He also swore at his wife and called her names. If he became angry about something while his wife was at work (e.g., a bill arrived in the mail), he would call and berate her. Embarrassed by his angry outbursts, he had recently begun to curtail his activities with the children, because keeping them at home was one way to prevent him from losing control in public. Although he had never been physically aggressive with his children (a report his wife confirmed), he had intrusive images of dramatic violence when he was angry with them, for example, recurrent images of himself hurling the children off the balcony. He found these violent images abhorrent and believed that they indicated he was a "monster" and a "horrible, sick person."

In addition to his difficulty managing his anger, Xavier complained of other symptoms of depression, including dysphoria, diminished sexual interest, difficulty maintaining a consistent sleep schedule, and weight gain. Xavier also spent quite a bit of time worrying about finances and work, and he was having a difficult time in his roles as father and husband. Xavier and his therapist agreed that his difficulty managing anger was the most important issue, because it affected all members of his family. Furthermore, improving his ability to manage anger had the potential to enact positive change on several other items on his Problem List, specifically those relating to the demands of parenthood and Xavier's relationship with his wife. Xavier also appeared ready to attempt change in this area of his life; he felt a growing acceptance of personal responsibility for his anger and its consequences. (See Figure 7.2 for Xavier's initial Problem List.)

Thus, the therapist decided that the first phase of treatment should focus on Xavier's anger, a high priority problem in which improvement could positively impact other areas of his life. In her discussions with Xavier about the Treatment Plan, his therapist explained why she believed it would be most fruitful to focus on his anger at the outset of treatment. Although she expected that helping Xavier to handle his anger would have positive effects on his depression and intermittent marital dissatisfaction, she also assured him that these problems would be addressed directly in subsequent phases of treatment, if necessary. Xavier and his therapist also agreed to review the Problem List after each phase of treatment to revise it, if necessary.

Xavier's description of his anger problems led his therapist initially to conceptualize them as being due to ineffective stress management and inappropriate assertiveness skills. Xavier described a pattern of mounting resentment against those with whom he disagreed but

	Client endorsed?
1. Frequent yelling at his children and wife	√
2. Calling his wife names	√
3. Keeping the children at home	√
4. Stonewalling wife	√
5. Nasty phone calls to wife at work	√
6. Negative appraisal of intrusive anger-related images	
7. Depressed mood	√
8. Not enough fun	
9. Decreased sexual interest	√
10. Weight gain	√
11. Generally high level of worry about finances and work	√
12. Difficulty coping with the demands of parenthood	√
13. Intermittent discontent with marital relationship	√

FIGURE 7.2. Xavier's initial Problem List.

chose not to confront (e.g., a supervisor or Xavier's wife). Moreover, he had some difficulty modulating his general arousal level; he said he felt like he had a "short fuse" and reacted intensely at "unpredictable" times. Based on both her conceptualization and on a review of the somewhat spotty treatment literature on anger management, the therapist chose an initial treatment approach that emphasized stress management and the development of assertiveness skills (see Figure 7.3).

Assessment Plan

Because the main goal of the initial phase of treatment was to reduce the frequency of angry outbursts toward his wife and children, Xavier completed daily records of his anger outbursts (see Figure 7.4). "Anger outbursts" were operationally defined as incidents in which Xavier raised his voice above his usual level for more than 60 seconds, something that he and his wife both indicated he did only when angry. Xavier's daily record sheet also included columns for recording the triggers to his anger, as well as describing his thoughts related to each episode. The therapist included a column for Xavier's angry behavior

Treatment Phase I	Date: 1/05/00

Aims: **1.** Reduce frequency of yelling at children and wife.

            2. Stop name-calling, and stop calling wife at work when angry.

            3. Express desires assertively before letting anger build.

Measures: **1.** Daily record of anger outbursts (self-report)
(attach graph)
            2. Daily record of anger outbursts (wife's report)

            3. Beck Depression Inventory (every 3 weeks)

Strategies: **1.** Identify anger triggers.

            2. Assertiveness skills training

            3. Relaxation and breathing training for stress management

            4. Encourage proactive use of stress management and assertiveness in situations that usually trigger anger.

Date for Phase I Progress Review: Session 12 (estimated 3/23/00)

FIGURE 7.3. Xavier's initial Treatment Plan: Phase I.

because several of the aims for this treatment phase were related to behaviors such as yelling or name-calling. Xavier agreed that his wife might have some insight to offer on his anger outbursts, and he wanted to begin talking with his wife about his problem with anger. Accordingly, the therapist created a similar record of Xavier's anger outbursts for his wife to complete. His wife's form did not contain a column for thoughts, but more space was allotted for describing Xavier's angry behavior.

Although the treatment strategies in Phase I were directed toward helping Xavier manage his anger, his therapist was also concerned about his depression, so she asked him to complete a Beck Depression Inventory (BDI) every 3 weeks as a continuing assessment. Although she did not necessarily expect to see a reduction in his depression, she felt more comfortable leaving Xavier's depression temporarily on the back burner of her treatment approach as long as she assessed it regularly. Had the depression escalated considerably during Phase I, the therapist would have considered switching to a new therapy phase to manage this emergent problem.

Date	Severity (0–10)	Angry behavior	What was the situation? With whom were you angry?	Thoughts before and during the outburst
11/2	6	Yelling, name calling	My wife came home late and the dinner I cooked was cold—angry with her.	She doesn't care about me or our family. She thinks I'm a bad husband.
11/3	5	Yelling	The supervisor didn't like my work—angry with self.	I'm a failure.
	7	Yelling	Wife critical of me—angry with her.	I'm useless, incompetent.
11/4	0		No outbursts today.	
11/5	4	Yelling	Son was slow in getting ready for school—angry with him.	He's making us late on purpose. I don't have any authority as a father.
11/6	9	Stonewalling	Wife critical and demanding—angry with her.	She doesn't have faith in me. Our marriage is doomed.
11/7	0		No outbursts today.	
11/8	3	Yelling	Son making noise while I was working—angry with him.	I can't control my son. I'm a bad father.

FIGURE 7.4. Daily Record of Xavier's anger outbursts.

179

Establishing a Baseline

Because of impending holidays and a cancelled session, 2 weeks elapsed between the initial evaluation and the first treatment session. Xavier's therapist had given him anger records during the intake session, and he and his wife completed these daily records during the 2 weeks before his first session to determine a baseline for his outbursts. Figure 7.5 shows this baseline (marked as session "0"), with acceptable agreement between Xavier's and his wife's daily records. Xavier and his therapist agreed on a treatment goal for Phase I of two or fewer anger outbursts per week. Xavier also completed a BDI during this time, obtaining a baseline score of 26, which supported the therapist's impression of the need to monitor his depression on a regular basis (see Figure 7.6).

Treatment

The therapist's first goal was to help Xavier identify triggers that provoked his rage. This strategy served as an assessment as well as an intervention in the sense that the therapist came to better understand Xavier's pattern of anger; at the same time, Xavier learned to spot anger triggers earlier in the rage-escalation process. Due to her conceptualization of Xavier's anger problems, the therapist then worked with Xavier to develop and practice appropriate assertiveness (through role plays and homework assignments). She also taught relaxation skills to

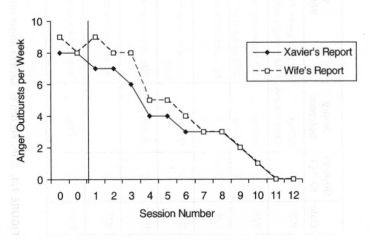

FIGURE 7.5. Xavier's anger outbursts during Treatment Phase I

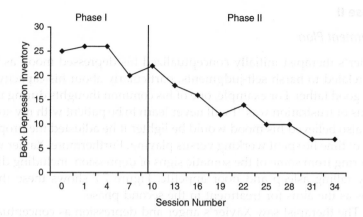

FIGURE 7.6. Xavier's change in BDI score over Treatment Phases I and II

Xavier and encouraged him to practice them daily. These strategies were aimed at providing him with adaptive skills to address frustrating or irritating situations as well as to help him calm himself when he became more aroused than the circumstances warranted. The therapist's final strategy was to help Xavier apply these strategies appropriately and solve problems he encountered in using the strategies.

Progress Review

Xavier's therapist tracked his anger outbursts (as reported by both Xavier and his wife) weekly throughout the first phase of treatment, which lasted for 12 sessions before the first planned Progress Review. Although the therapist attended to the full array of information contained in the anger records, she focused on the frequency of outbursts for the formal graphed data she shared with Xavier. Their discussion during the Progress Review also covered changes in more qualitative aspects of the anger records. As indicated in Figure 7.5, Xavier experienced a marked decrease in the frequency of his anger outbursts during this time, and his wife's report corroborated this observation.

Xavier also completed a BDI every 3 weeks. Figure 7.6 shows that Xavier's depression remained relatively steady during the first phase, in spite of his success at managing his anger. Xavier and his therapist agreed that his depression remained a considerable problem. Accordingly, his therapist prepared to begin addressing his depression in the second phase of therapy.

Phase II

Treatment Plan

Xavier's therapist initially conceptualized his depressed mood as being related to harsh self-judgments, particularly about his capacity to be a good father. For example, one of his common thoughts during moments of frustration was "I will never learn to be patient with my son." She also believed his mood would be lighter if he adjusted the proportion of time he spent working versus playing. Furthermore, Xavier was suffering from some of the somatic signs of depression, including difficulty falling asleep and poor appetite. Figure 7.7 shows these three areas as the aims for treatment in the second phase.

The therapist saw Xavier's anger and depression as conceptually linked, because some of the cognitions he reported during anger-evoking situations were similar to those he reported during times of low mood. One example was related to his intrusive violent images. Although many people experience aggressive images during times of anger, Xavier judged himself very harshly in response to these unbidden images, believing they provided evidence that he was a terrible person. For him, having a mental image of hitting someone was as bad as actually doing it. Reviewing the case conceptualization, along with

Treatment Phase II	**Date:** *4/05/00*
Aims:	**1.** Reduce believability of depressive cognitions (e.g., I will never be a good parent).
	2. Normalize sleep patterns and appetite.
	3. Increase proportion of leisure versus work time.
Measures: *(attach graph)*	**1.** Beck Depression Inventory (every 3 weeks)
	2. Diary of daily events (including pleasant activities and work)
Strategies:	**1.** Cognitive restructuring in conjunction with thought records (e.g., challenge all-or-none thinking with inquiries about evidence).
	2. Send for pharmacological consultation.
	3. Behavioral contracting (e.g., engage in pleasure reading for 30 minutes a day).
Date for Phase II Progress Review: Session 12 (estimated 6/28/00)	

FIGURE 7.7. Xavier's initial Treatment Plan: Phase II.

the empirical literature, led the therapist to plan a cognitive-behavioral approach toward Xavier's depression. She chose this approach because it is a well-researched treatment for depression. Furthermore, Xavier had responded well to a structured approach in the first phase of treatment, and he was able to report and discuss his thoughts with relative ease. Finally, in response to Xavier's request, she arranged a pharmacological consultation, and Xavier began taking Zoloft to further manage his depressive symptoms and assist him with impulse control. Note that because Xavier began pharmacological and psychological treatments at the same time in Phase II, the therapist would not be able to tell which intervention was responsible for any observed improvement.

Assessing Progress

Xavier continued to complete the BDI every 3 weeks in the second phase of treatment. His therapist viewed the BDI as a reliable and valid instrument that would assess not only his sleep and appetite problems but also his affective and cognitive symptoms of depression. Because one aim was for Xavier to have more fun, the therapist asked him to keep a diary of his daily activities, so they could review together the amount of time he spent in pleasant activities compared to chores or work. Xavier also continued to monitor his thoughts during difficult situations, as he had during Phase I (e.g., Figure 7.7), but this time he focused on his thoughts during times of low mood rather than anger.

Over the course of treatment, as indicated by Figure 7.6, Xavier's overall level of depression dropped to the normal range. During the first few weeks of this phase of treatment, Xavier successfully kept a diary of his daily activities, but he soon found this assessment strategy to be burdensome. When his therapist noticed Xavier's noncompliance with the diary, she considered some of the potential obstacles noted in the Decision Tree. She hypothesized that the diary provided too little reward for the time involved in completing it. Therefore, she changed strategies and used part of the session time to help Xavier plan at least one pleasant event each day. She made note of these plans and asked him about each pleasant event at the subsequent session. Although her initial assessment strategy had failed, this alternate plan enabled her to obtain sufficient information about Xavier's leisure activities to evaluate his progress on that aim.

Xavier and his therapist agreed that the improvement in his depression and the maintenance of improved ability to manage his anger signaled the end of Phase II. When he and his therapist reviewed the

Problem List, they agreed that his progress on items 11 (worry about money and work) and 12 (difficulty coping with parenthood) had improved such that these items did not require specific intervention.

At this time, Xavier and his therapist ended therapy. Although his marital discontent was still an issue, Xavier wanted to try to work things out for himself in the relationship. He felt he had made many changes in the previous months of therapy, and he believed the relationship needed some time to adjust to his new ways of managing his mood.

Phase III

Six months later, Xavier again sought a brief course of therapy to help him resolve his ambivalence about remaining in his marriage. His wife was dealing with some emotional issues of her own, and the couple had been arguing frequently, even though Xavier maintained that his anger outbursts and depression were not current problems. The main issues were disagreements over financial concerns and parenting. For example, Xavier wanted to enroll the children in community sports, but his wife believed the children had too many afterschool activities. The couple also frequently argued about how involved the children should be in their church. They reported that they did not communicate well with each other—each feeling that the other was too bossy. Their sexual relationship had been nonexistent for months due to the tension between them. Xavier felt hopeless about their ability to resolve these problems, and he was deeply ambivalent about whether to remain in the marriage.

Treatment Plan

Xavier's marital distress was approached initially within an individual-treatment context, mainly because he wished to explore his ambivalence about remaining in the marriage without his wife being present. To help Xavier explore his reasons for remaining in versus leaving the marriage, his therapist tentatively planned a motivational interviewing approach for Phase III. She saw this as essentially a brief exploratory phase in which she helped Xavier to clarify his aims. She left open the possibility of communication training with Xavier's wife during later conjoint sessions (as indicated in parentheses in the Treatment Plan for Phase III; see Figure 7.8).

Xavier's main aims in Phase III were to resolve his ambivalence about remaining in the marriage and, if he remained, to reduce the level of discord in the marriage. At first, Xavier was unable to express

Treatment Phase III	Date: 1/24/01
Aims:	**1.** Resolve ambivalence about remaining in marriage.
	2. Reduce marital discord.
Measures:	**1.** Dyadic Adjustment Scale
(attach graph)	**2.** Daily diary of satisfaction with marital interactions
Strategies:	**1.** Motivational interviewing with client
	2. (Communication training with client and wife)
Date for Phase III Progress Review:	Session 12 (estimated 4/10/01)

FIGURE 7.8. Xavier's Treatment Plan: Tentative Phase III.

exactly how the marriage was dissatisfying to him, except to say that he and his wife argued too frequently and that their intimacy was gone. As the therapist helped Xavier to specify the problems in his marriage and to envision how he would like things to be, Xavier began to feel hopeful that he wanted the marriage to work.

Using a motivational interviewing approach, the psychologist helped Xavier to ascertain his level of commitment to the marriage and his willingness to work on improving it. After three sessions of discussing these issues, Xavier had regained some optimism and gained a clearer sense of his own wishes related to the marriage. He decided he wanted to work on the relationship rather than leave it. Accordingly, the therapist ended the Phase III intervention and referred Xavier and his wife to a couple therapist.

Phase IV

A year later, Xavier returned to therapy with his original psychologist. He had again begun to experience occasional anger outbursts, so he sought some booster sessions to reinforce the anger management and assertiveness skills he had learned in Phase I. A more important concern was he had begun to question his deep involvement with the Seventh Day Adventist Church and had developed a related desire to pursue spiritual growth in other areas. Because he had been deeply involved with the Church for many years, his sense of self was partly defined by his religion and spirituality. Nevertheless, Xavier had begun to feel a spiritual void, about which he felt conflicted and confused.

Problem List and Treatment Plan

Because it had been so long since he had last been in therapy, Xavier and his therapist first reviewed his original Problem List. Most of his old problems with anger had not resurfaced, but Xavier had noticed he was yelling more often at his wife and children. He worried he might be slipping into his old anger patterns. Depression was also not a current problem, nor was worry or coping with fatherhood. Xavier added new problems to the list—problems of a more existential nature. Now that his children were getting older, Xavier had begun to experience an emptiness and pointlessness that he related to spirituality. He felt guilty about expressing any feelings of discontent with the Church. The therapist developed a new Treatment Plan that included a review of some elements that had been helpful during Phase I plus some components with a humanistic inquiry approach (see Figure 7.9). The fourth phase of treatment thus began with a review of assertiveness and relaxation skills, with role-playing and homework assignments to practice skills and monitor progress.

Treatment Phase IV   Date: 3/14/02

Aims: **1.** Regain sense of control over anger at home.

        2. Reduce ambivalence and guilt related to Church.

        3. Identify new areas of spirituality that are not encompassed by Church teachings.

Measures: **1.** Diary of anger outbursts
(attach graph)
        2. Diary of spiritual activities inside and outside of Church

        3. Daily Spiritual Experiences (DSE) scale (every 2 weeks)

Strategies: **1.** Reinforce cognitive coping and anger management skills.

        2. Humanistic inquiry into acceptable paths for spiritual growth.

        3. Assign homework of engaging in new activities for spiritual growth.

Date for Phase IV Progress Review: Session 8 (estimated 5/9/02)

FIGURE 7.9. Xavier's Treatment Plan: Phase IV.

Treatment

The therapist first helped Xavier to clarify what level of involvement with his church was acceptable to him, then helped him to identify and pursue new areas of spiritual stimulation and growth. Assessment in this domain was accomplished with a weekly record of activities or events that Xavier said he experienced in a spiritual way. The purpose of the weekly diary was to help him better identify what he meant by "spiritual." Xavier also completed the short form (5 items) of the Daily Spiritual Experiences (DES) scale. The full (long form) version of this scale is included in the Appendix, but the therapist used the short form because she felt that its questions adequately addressed several aspects of Xavier's spiritual search. More details on the Daily Spiritual Experiences scale can be obtained in Underwood (1999).

Progress Review

At the Phase IV Progress Review, the therapist observed that Xavier had regained control over his anger outbursts. Although he had been yelling at his wife or children about twice a week when he began Phase IV, by the end of the phase, his diary often indicated several weeks between outbursts. As Xavier had become clearer in his own mind about what spirituality meant for him, he accordingly became less ambivalent about his Church. Although it was a difficult decision for him, he ultimately decided to be involved less formally in its activities. He developed and pursued several other avenues of his own spiritual growth that better fit with his current needs and desires. Figure 7.10 presents the change in Xavier's score on the DSE scale over this fourth phase of treatment.

Xavier's case illustrates some of the easier and more challenging aspects of using the PACC method. His first two treatment phases involved fairly straightforward emotional problems (i.e., depression and anger), for which numerous assessment tools have been developed. Although he was reasonably compliant with assessment, Xavier was unable to follow through on one of the self-monitoring assignments during Phase II, and his therapist had to reconsider how to assess his engagement in pleasant activities. Phase III was cut short (with his individual therapist) because Xavier decided to accept a referral to couple therapy to address his aims related to his marriage. Phase IV involved therapy for a problem with spirituality, which posed difficulties for the therapist and Xavier in conceptual-

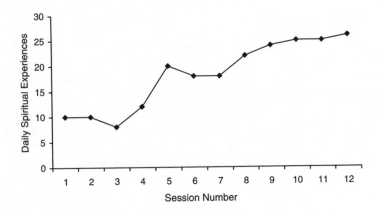

FIGURE 7.10. Xavier's Daily Spiritual Experiences.

ization, aims, and measurement. Having illustrated the course of one client's treatment within the PACC system, we now turn to relevant ethical considerations.

ETHICAL IMPLICATIONS OF USING PACC

Using the PACC approach in clinical practice touches on several important ethical concerns, including those involved with confidentiality, informed consent, record keeping, and scope of practice. We begin a discussion of these issues here, although ethical conflicts arise in highly idiosyncratic situations, and it is often helpful to seek supervision or consultation with a colleague before deciding on a course of action.

Confidentiality and Collateral Informants

An ideal plan for comprehensive assessment may involve obtaining information from individuals other than the client, as was the case with Xavier's wife, who provided a second viewpoint on the frequency of his anger episodes. Collateral informants are commonly used when working with children (e.g., teacher or parent reports), but they are used relatively rarely for adult clients. Recruiting a loved one to help with assessment can have clear benefits, because some clients are unable to report certain types of information if they are insufficiently aware of their own behavior. Xavier's own accounting of the frequency of his anger outbursts was very consistent with his wife's report, but the therapist initially asked Xavier's wife to keep a separate rating form, because shame about uncontrolled anger outbursts seemed to create the potential for him to minimize the problem. Although Xavier was initially puzzled when his therapist suggested he and his wife separately monitor his anger outbursts, he agreed that his wife might notice them more reliably than he would.

In considering whether to use a collateral informant, the therapist should first carefully consider the trade-off between the potential value of the information and the risks associated with the somewhat diminished confidentiality involved in obtaining information from another person. For example, therapists would ordinarily refrain from asking a client's children for any information about him or her. However, in the case of an elderly client who has had some difficulties in maintaining ordinary activities of daily living, occasional reports from adult children may be warranted on important issues, such as whether the client has food in the refrigerator.

If, after a careful consideration of the risks and potential benefits, the therapist believes that a collateral informant would be appropriate, he or she must then clearly explain this trade-off to the client, so she or he can make a decision about it. This discussion should include acknowledgment of the ways that confidentiality will be compromised by the involvement of others and an indication of the potential utility of the information others will provide. The clinician should also clearly outline the limits of any information that will be shared with those who help with assessment (e.g., how the therapist will respond to questions from the collateral informant). After a discussion of all these issues, the client will be in a position to provide or decline informed consent (discussed in the upcoming section) for the use of collateral informants. Obviously, the client's wishes about confidentiality must be respected even if the therapist believes collateral information is important (although the power to withhold consent is sometimes altered in forensic or institutional settings).

Collaboration and Informed Consent in the Therapeutic Relationship

As we discussed in earlier chapters, the degree of collaboration between a therapist and client depends on factors related to the therapist, the client, and the presenting problem. When therapists are generating a Problem List or thinking ahead about potential phases of treatment, they may choose not to share all of their ideas with their clients. Although we generally advocate a straightforward approach with clients, we do recognize some instances in which the best strategy is not a fully collaborative one. An example illustrates one such situation from our own practice.

Ezekiel, a 52-year-old man, sought treatment for long-standing depression and social isolation. During the initial evaluation, his therapist became concerned about the extent of his alcohol use, which appeared to be excessive and maladaptive. Ezekiel, however, was very defensive when discussing his alcohol use, because his father had been an alcoholic with a violent temper. Although his therapist considered Ezekiel's alcohol use to be a problem that probably contributed to maintaining his depression, she chose not to share her view of this problem right away. Instead, she raised the issue of alcohol use in casual, conversational moments to keep tabs on it during the first two phases of treatment. After they had worked on Ezekiel's presenting complaints of depression and social isolation, the therapeutic relationship was very solid, and the therapist directly raised her concerns about his use of alcohol. Ezekiel agreed to monitor his alcohol use for several weeks to evaluate how much he was using and the situations in which he chose to drink. Faced with these data, Ezekiel and his therapist then collaboratively formulated treatment goals for the third (final) phase of treatment.

The issue of how much and what kind of feedback to give to clients is a controversial point of ethics that must be examined continually for each client. In our view, the therapist should provide all pertinent information for the client to engage in informed consent; that is, the client should know the aims of treatment, how progress toward the aims will be measured, and the rough outline of the planned therapeutic strategies. Without this information, consent is not really "informed." However, we also regard each phase of treatment as a new occasion for obtaining informed consent; we see our clients as consenting to specific phases of treatment. At times, they will consent to the first phase or two but decline to engage in another phase, because their goals do not match the goals of the therapist. The PACC approach facilitates the explicit discussion of treatment goals in an ongoing way, but the onus is still on the therapist to balance professional opinions with explicit feedback to facilitate the client's participation in and consent for mental health care.

Scope of Practice

The phase model of the PACC approach lends itself nicely to compartmentalizing aspects of treatment for clients with complicated problems. Ethical standards clearly state that clinicians should stay within the bounds of their areas of training and level of competence, which naturally necessitates collaboration with colleagues who have different areas of expertise. The PACC approach can lend structure and guidance in cases in which a client should be referred for an episode of specialty care. By prioritizing items on the Problem List and thinking ahead about the planned phases of treatment, the primary clinician can coordinate care and systematize assessment even when the client is temporarily consulting with a specialist. Xavier's case is a good example of this concept. His therapist could see from the Problem List and initial treatment planning that a marital therapy consultation might be required at a future point. The therapist made preliminary arrangements for such a referral in advance. When Xavier ultimately agreed to enter couple therapy with his wife, his individual therapist provided the anger outburst assessment form to the couple's therapist to maintain continuous assessment of this important behavior. By structuring the treatment in terms of explicit phases, each addressing specified aims, Xavier's therapist felt confident in finding an appropriate time to discuss the issue of the marital relationship.

APPLICATIONS OF PACC

Our discussion of the PACC system has thus far been set in the context of clinical practice, and we would like to take the opportunity to outline explicitly some of the ways that the approach can contribute to other settings we have not previously addressed.

Mental Health Services in a Large Organization

The PACC approach could be a valuable and feasible addition to larger clinical practice settings. For example, Veteran's Administration (VA) hospitals already have a computerized system to list problems for each client who seeks services. The computerized record-keeping system requires that therapists add new problems to the list if they become an active focus of treatment. The VA also has experimented with mandatory entry of GAF (Global Assessment of Functioning) scores periodically as a client's computer records are accessed and updated. These procedures could be folded into the more comprehensive system of assessment comprised by PACC. It is possible that a computer program might be generated to guide therapists through the Decision Tree, to remind them of the need for Progress Review, and to prompt them regarding other aspects of the treatment planning process.

Large hospitals often serve as comprehensive care centers. As such, the PACC approach might facilitate professional communication and consultation regarding a client's improvement. In this sense, the use of PACC could promote coordinated care (the ostensible goal of some managed care organizations) without an overemphasis on controlling cost. Similarly, the PACC model facilitates documentation of the Problem List and multiple phases of treatment, which may enhance treatment in large training hospitals in which transfer of care occurs frequently. In such settings, it is often difficult to speak with past therapists when taking on one of their previous clients. Using the PACC approach, the client's prior work in therapy (both progress markers and failed attempts) would be easily conveyed to the new therapist.

Coordinated care is especially important for clients with multifaceted problems that require a variety of services from a whole team of professionals. For example, some VA hospitals have a home-based primary care (HBPC) program for veterans who have multiple problems but are homebound and unable to come to the hospital. An interdisciplinary team of health care professionals (e.g., primary care physician, occupational therapist, pharmacist, psychologist, social worker, dietician) usually provides the services under HBPC. Multidisciplinary teams like those of the HBPC are often required to create treatment plans as part of regular case conference meetings. However, there is typically no systematic or formal assessment to determine whether the treatment plan is actually working. The PACC approach represents a structured system to facilitate this type of quality-of-care assessment in interdisciplinary team meetings.

Clinical Research

The PACC approach is designed to bridge the tools and philosophy of clinical science with the reality of clinical practice. We did not design the approach with clinical research in mind, but clinicians interested in becoming more involved in research can certainly use these tools to get started. By keeping track of the specific strategies used in treatment, as well as the outcomes of those strategies, clinicians are in an optimal position to gather initial data to support the utility of novel treatment approaches or to document specific types of clients who do not appear to respond to well-established treatment approaches. A documented set of clinical experiences is more credible than undocumented clinical lore when communicating with colleagues in formal settings such as conference symposia, books, and journal articles. Furthermore, for those practitioners interested in making a large commitment to research, systematic data can provide the necessary pilot work to support a successful grant application to test clinical hypotheses more stringently.

Doing large-scale research in a clinical setting is an enormous challenge, which is probably why most research of this type is done in university laboratory settings. Nevertheless, the field desperately needs more information about how treatments tested in those laboratories actually work in practice, where the clinicians, clients, and environments are heterogeneous. The solo practitioner probably cannot conduct research of this type, but it may be workable in a group practice or mental health clinic. In order to focus on a research question, it is wise to choose an area of the practice that is relatively homogenous, such as the "Adolescent Treatment Team" or "Substance Abuse Unit," then choose some measures that will be pertinent to nearly every client seen in the setting. We suggested some general measures in Chapter 4 (some which are included in the Appendix), but every area of practice has its own reliable and valid measures. The PACC system allows the practitioner to use a general measure for everyone, in addition to some measures that target particular issues for each client.

With this two-tiered measurement system, one can simultaneously gather data to compare across clients and data that are important for each individual client. The potential research questions in such a setting are broad, although some safeguards should be taken. For example, if an organization wanted to compare the outcomes of supervisees at various levels of training (e.g., second-year social work student, psychiatry resident, psychology intern, postdoctoral fellow), it would be important to control for the fact that more difficult cases may be assigned to supervisees with greater training. If random assignment of cases to the supervisees is unacceptable, then one must allow for some adjustment on the basis of difficulty of caseload when analyzing and interpreting the results. Research on such questions can make an important contribution to the literature, but the added experimental control and manipulations required to make causal inferences are prohibitive in most practice settings.

Publishing case studies also raises important ethical questions related to our earlier discussion of informed consent. In general, a clinician would not seek an Institutional Review Board (IRB) review for data collected in the context of normal clinical practice, such as internal quality assurance projects. Collecting data for research purposes does generally require an IRB review and informed consent from the study participants. If a practitioner knows in advance that he or she wants to publish data, then it would be better to seek IRB approval and informed consent from the client. In contrast, if the clinician decides later to publish the case information, then the use of the client's data may be considered a chart review, for which most IRBs have established procedures and safeguards. We recommend that clinicians consult their local IRB if they are in an academic or medical setting, or their practice manager, if they work in private or group practice, to determine if a policy for evaluating measures and publishing case material exists. The guidelines are usually not prohibitively restrictive, and we encourage clinicians to consider taking advantage of the material collected when using the PACC approach to advance dissemination of single-case design studies.

Comparisons across Clients

Comparing a client's data across different points in time is natural in the PACC approach given the goal of monitoring treatment with ongoing assessment. However, it may also be helpful to compare across clients, therapists, or treatment sites, perhaps for research purposes or to evaluate "best practices." In such cases, it is helpful to convert clients' pre- and posttreatment scores to norms, such as percentiles, Z scores, or T scores. The basic rudiments of normative data are available for a wide variety of assessment tools, usually published in the scoring manuals or journal articles in which the measure was initially introduced. Clients' scores can be compared to the published results from other clients with the same problem or to clients with no psychological complaints. Comparing clients' scores with norms is useful for defining a numerical goal for treatment (e.g., one standard deviation below the mean for a normal sample) or even for simply understanding the degree of impairment shown by the clients (before or even after treatment). For information on how to perform these statistical conversions, the interested reader can consult any introductory statistics text-book for the social sciences.

When comparing data across clients, one caveat is warranted: One cannot assume that the same assessment tool will result in comparable information if administered under different circumstances. Extensive evidence illustrates that behavior tends to be situation-specific (Mischel, 1968), so evaluation across people or time requires similar testing circumstances. To use an obvious example, asking a child about her hitting behaviors when she is alone will likely yield different responses than asking the child the same question when her parent or teacher is in the room. An entertaining but compelling example of this discrepancy comes from the classic studies by Hartshorne and May (1928), who demonstrated that children's honesty varies greatly depending on whether the situation occurs at home, in the classroom, at a party, or during an athletic contest. Such concerns are applicable to adults as well as to children.

Clinical Training and Teaching

The PACC model is ideal for providing structure for students who are just beginning to learn to do treatment planning. New therapists often get caught up in the client's sense of being overwhelmed by problems, and creating a Problem List can help new therapists feel they are at least keeping tabs on all of the important issues (even if the issues cannot be addressed all at once). When working with students (who are new to doing therapy), we encourage supervisors to provide concrete examples of the elements to include in the first phase of the Treatment Plan (i.e., lists of potential aims, measures, and strategies). As students' skills develop, they will be able to prepare more of the elements of the Treatment Plan in advance of a supervisory session, and the aims, strategies, and measures can be discussed during supervision. Because the PACC system makes concrete the steps that many clinicians implicitly use for treatment planning, students benefit from having those steps made explicit.

We find that students often need guidance in developing aims that are specific enough for the given phase of treatment. Often, students are tempted to use aims that are better conceptualized as overall goals for the client. When working with students, we tend to focus on smaller segments of treatment in order to provide structure. For example, a professional clinician might consider Xavier's treatment to consist of four phases, roughly characterized as anger, depression, marriage, and spirituality. Each treatment phase might encompass many weeks in a long-term treatment. We encourage students to be as specific as possible about the aims, measures, and strategies. In some cases, this specificity might involve conceptualizing the treatment as consisting of more phases, each targeting a more specific goal. In this event, the measures may not change across several phases.

For example, Xavier's Phase I could have involved several smaller phases that represent each of the strategies. Each of the strategies listed in Figure 7.3 is naturally composed of many smaller interventions, and beginning students often benefit from explicitly outlining these smaller interventions. Rather than the overall aim of reducing uncontrolled anger at family members, an appropriate aim for an advanced student or professional, the newer therapist may articulate aims of (1) recognizing and anticipating anger-evoking situations, (2) learning to express wants and needs assertively, (3) learning how to deescalate the intensity of his emotion, and (4) developing the ability to calm down in frustrating and irritating situations. These more specific aims can be grouped as appropriate to form smaller treatment phases to help students maintain focus. The daily record of anger outbursts would still be collected from Xavier and his wife, and would provide continuity between the more numerous phases.

Business Implications of PACC

Recent downward pressures on pricing and availability of mental health care have been distressing to many mental health professionals. Bartlett (1997) reported price drops of 30–40% in the mid-1990s in the commercial carve-out area of the behavioral health care marketplace, which means that far less money is available to provide mental health services when they are separated from other health care. In this climate of intense competition, third-party insurers rely increasingly on assessments of treatment efficacy to make decisions about coverage (O'Keefe et al., 1996). This trend may at first sound alarming, because many mental health care practitioners have not directed explicit attention toward quality and outcomes. However, we believe it is better than basing decisions on price alone. Meaningfully defining and measuring quality of care may begin to lead the market toward coverage decisions based on value (the relationship of cost and quality) rather than cost alone (Bartlett, 1997).

The American Psychiatric Association (1997) already encourages purchasers of mental health contracts to incorporate performance indicators, such as administrative proficiency, financial performance, and cost-shifting considerations, into those contracts. Other indicators of good performance include client satisfaction and "clinical quality." Clinical quality in this case refers to markers such as recidivism and relapse rates, lag time between the end of acute treatment and contact with community-based care, and improved quality of life and functioning.

As Barlett (1997) outlined, the challenge in using performance indicators is to resolve the technical, organizational, and cultural obstacles to defining and measuring quality. The PACC model provides recommendations that help to address some of the technical questions, and other books on measuring outcomes in mental health have addressed organizational and cultural obstacles (Lyons, Howard, O'Mahoney, & Lish, 1997; Ogles, Lambert, & Masters, 1996; Sederer & Dickey, 1996). Although PACC is directed toward the individual clinician who wishes to use measurement of outcomes to improve accountability and confidence in treatment planning, the same principles can easily be applied within a group of clinicians who share the same goals. Thus, even though PACC is designed at the individual client level, these results can be aggregated to reflect performance outcomes within and across treatment settings.

Measuring quality of care opens up many possibilities beyond guiding treatment planning for individual clients. For example, some quality-of-care models include best practices or benchmarking, in which the most successful clinicians (with a given client population) are identified, and other clinicians learn intervention strategies from those providers. Quantifying the outcomes of treatment is one way to ensure that service improvements are based on clients' needs rather than cost considerations or administrative requirements alone. This client-centered focus is an element of the total quality management approach, which is a business philosophy that has helpful applications to service provision in mental health care (Forquer & Muse, 1996).

The stepped care models of psychotherapy illustrate another application that follows from measuring outcomes. These models seek to maximize efficient allocation of resources by tailoring the level of intervention to the needs of the client. Clients who require long-term care from a highly trained specialist receive different services than clients who are likely to benefit from self-help materials or a brief psychoeducational group conducted by a paraprofessional (Haaga, 2000). The premise is that lower cost interventions are tried first, with more intensive approaches reserved for those who do not improve sufficiently during the initial intervention. Obviously, good identification and measurement of the client's problems are essential to feel confident about treatment allocation in stepped care models.

Furthermore, as mental health care moves toward capitated systems that are more fully integrated within the rest of health care, there will be an even greater need to monitor clients' progress so that relapse rates are minimized. Because most people with mental health problems remain untreated, Keisler (2000) argues that mental health professionals must consider the issue of "good-enough treatment." The "good-enough" concept implies that treatment should be no more than "sufficient" to avoid relapse and return to care, because providing everyone with "ideal" treatment would be prohibitively expensive. Naturally, we all wish for resources to help clients reach their fullest potential, but this is not possible in the real world. The PACC system of treatment planning has the potential to help practitioners manage some of these trade-offs by making goals and measurement explicit.

FINAL COMMENTS

In developing the PACC system, we initially aimed to provide tools for clinicians practicing in settings that do not lend themselves to the use of manualized, empirically supported treatments. For example, some populations (e.g., Native American or First Nations communities) or problem areas (e.g., spousal abuse) have not been studied sufficiently to have well-established treatments. PACC provides a system for using evidence-based practice when the research literature does not provide adequate guidance for treatment planning with a given client. Evidence-based practice can still be used if "evidence" also includes data the clinician collects to document the effects of intervention. Throughout this book, we have described ways that these procedures—explicitly defining treatment aims, measuring progress toward those aims in reliable and valid ways, and continually reevaluating the treatment plan in light of the data—can boost the quality and perhaps the cost-effectiveness of treatment.

In an ideal world, gathering systematic data can provide managers and decision makers with more accurate information for organizational planning. The PACC system can help to build good databases to address important questions, such as how long it generally takes to achieve certain mental health goals. The first step is for frontline service providers in psychology, social work, and psychiatry to implement evidence-based practices seriously. After that, we can start to insist that managed care organizations and other decision makers also rely on evidence-based practices for broader decisions about mental health care coverage.

For experienced clinicians, the PACC system helps make explicit many of the treatment planning practices that are likely standard practice, adding the concept of ongoing measurement. For new therapists, following the PACC model can help organize the approach to treatment and ensure conscientious and efficient clinical practice. By formulating a problem list that comprehensively evaluates functioning across a range of biopsychosocial domains, clinicians are less likely to miss an important problem or be unaware of potential therapy-interfering circumstances. Once this list has been prioritized, the client and therapist collaboratively develop a Treatment Plan, with specified aims, strategies, and measures to evaluate progress. Using client data to regularly review progress increases motivation for further gains and prevents an ineffective therapy from continuing unchecked. Our hope is that the PACC system can respond to the diverse challenges of practicing mental health care in the 21st century to provide clinicians with a flexible approach to therapy that takes advantage of the treatment outcome literature and also responds to clients' unique needs.

MEASURES
FOR TRACKING
CLIENTS' PROGRESS

CONTENTS

OVERVIEW

The items in this Appendix are intended to help clinicians get started in the measurement of their clients' progress. Given the difficulty of accessing measures, we have reprinted some measures and provided information for how to access others. These measures were selected because they are useful for tracking progress during a given treatment phase (i.e., they are sensitive to change), they are brief and easy to administer, and they have adequate psychometric properties.

These measures do not cover the entire range of psychological problems, due to space constraints, but are all measures of common disorders or adjustment issues likely to be encountered in everyday clinical practice. In addition to measures of anxiety and mood, we have included measures of self-esteem, eating disorders, psychosis, and marital satisfaction. Given that a Problem List may include issues that occur across a range of biopsychosocial domains, we have also included measures of spirituality and acculturation. Finally, because a measurement plan ideally incorporates both global and specific measures, the Brief Psychiatric Rating Scale is reprinted to serve as a broad measure of psychiatric functioning.

We begin with a brief description of each instrument and the population for which it is appropriate, and also provide scoring information and group norms where possible. We have also reprinted the instruments for which we were able to get permission. As mentioned, this Appendix is designed as a starting point. There are many excellent additional resources available that contain multiple instruments related to specific clinical populations of interest and unique assessment needs. Chapter 4 includes a list of such resources that clinicians may consider purchasing, or alternatively, many of these resources are available at academic libraries.

DESCRIPTION OF THE MEASURES

Brief Psychiatric Rating Scale

The BPRS, useful as a global measure of functioning for more severely ill populations, is composed of a series of primary symptom dimensions (e.g., depression, hostility, and psychoticism), as well as a global pathology index. Thus, it can be used as an overall index, or clinicians may choose to focus on only those dimensions that are relevant to their clients for ongoing progress evaluation. Please see Rhoades and Overall (1988) for helpful sample questions to guide the interviewer, because each item is associated with a definition that is necessary to make reliable and valid ratings.

As a comparison point, Adams, Palmer, Crook, and O'Brien (2000) examined BPRS ratings for 89 patients on admission to an acute psychiatric ward. The primary diagnoses included affective disorders (35%), drug/alcohol abuse (36%), psychosis (16%), and personality disorders (11%). The *mean* score was 22.5 (*SD* = 13.6), comparable with levels found in other studies. The scores were particularly high for those with psychosis, *M* = 39.5 (*SD* = 15.5) and affective disorder, *M* = 24.0 (*SD* = 10.3).

Bulimia Test—Revised

The original Bulimia Test was revised to accommodate the DSM-III-R criteria of bulimia nervosa and is an effective tool for evaluating common symptoms of bulimia nervosa (both in initial diagnostic assessment and over the course of treatment). The BULIT-R, reproduced here, was revised to accommodate DSM-IV criteria for bulimia nervosa. The 36-item scale takes about 10 minutes to complete and has been found useful in measuring severity of bulimic symptoms and evaluating treatment outcome. Cross-validation was performed on independent samples of bulimic and college control subjects, and the BULIT-R predicted group membership well. The scale also has evidenced good test–retest reliability and construct validity.

Of the 36 items listed, 28 are used for the total score, and 8 items pertaining to weight control behavior are not tallied in the summary score. Items 6, 11, 19, 20, 27, 29, 31, and 36 are not scored. Items 1, 3 4, 9, 18, 22, 24, 25, 33, and 34 are scored in a forward scoring format in which 1 = 1 and 5 = 5. The remaining 18 items are reverse scored; choice 1 receives 5 points, and choice 5 receives 1 point. After rescaling the reverse scored items, the 28 items are totaled.

In two studies, mean scores for bulimic women were 117.9 and 118.1, whereas the means for nonclinical women were 57.5 and 59.6. The authors suggest an acceptable cutoff score for bulimia should be 104. Although this scale has good psychometric support, individuals with eating disorders are often secretive about their symptoms, often necessitating multiple symptom measures. Corroborating indicators (such as tracking frequency of binge episodes) are advised when using this measure.

Please note: The BULIT-R has been reproduced here with permission from Mark H. Thelen. Permission has *not* been granted for photocopying the measure from this book, but a copy of the BULIT-R, along with scoring information, may be obtained from Mark H. Thelen, Department of Psychology, University of Missouri–Columbia, 210 McAlester Hall, Columbia, MO 65211. The current cost is $80.00 for use in a single research project and $160.00 for unlimited use in an applied setting.

Center for Epidemiologic Studies—Depression Scale (CES-D)

One of the advantages of the CES-D measure for depression in adolescents and adults is that it has been used in both urban and rural populations, and in cross-cultural studies of depression. The 20-item measure was developed by researchers at the National Institute of Mental Health. There is no cost to use this scale.

Each depressive symptom is measured on a scale from 0 (rarely or none of the time) to 3 (most or all of the time), yielding a summed total score. The scores can range from 0 to 60. A score greater than 16 typically identifies people at risk for clinical depression in the United States (Radloff, 1977). Radloff reported means of 9.1 for community samples and 24.4 for one sample of patients. In North American samples, four factors emerge: depressive affect, somatic symptoms, positive affect, and interpersonal relations. The CES-D has been found to be a reliable measure of depression among European American, African American, and Mexican American groups (Golding & Burnam, 1990; Roberts, 1980). The cutoff score should perhaps be raised for some groups; Cho et al. (1993) reported the cutoff point that best predicted current major depression to be 17 for Cuban Americans and 20 for Puerto Ricans.

Daily Spiritual Experiences Scale

This scale is designed to be a relatively direct measure of day-to-day spiritual experiences of an ordinary person. Thus, it is designed to capture the impact of religion and spirituality on daily life and does not reflect more unusual experiences, such as near death or out of body events. We have found it an effective tool to monitor progress for clients who wish to change or simply reevaluate spirituality or their relationship with the divine.

The short form of this scale is items 1, 3, 8, and 11, plus a combination of items 4 and 5, "I feel God's love for me, directly or through others." The full report describing this measure can be obtained at *http://www.fetzer.org/resources/resources_multidimens.htm* or by writing to The Fetzer Institute at 9292 West KL Avenue, Kalamazoo, MI 49009-9398, or by calling (616) 375-2000.

Kansas Marital Satisfaction Scale

One of the primary advantages of this scale is that it is extremely brief and can be administered to both men and women. It assesses the level of satisfaction in marriage, so it can be an effective measure for ongoing evaluation in couple therapy. Within various Kansas communities, Schumm et al. (1986) reported mean scores of 17.9 (*SD* = 2.7) for husbands and 17.4 (*SD* = 3.2) for wives. There is no cost to use this scale.

Psychotic Symptoms Rating Scales

This scale has good psychometric properties and was designed to be comprehensive yet easy to administer. The 17-item questionnaire consists of two subscales that rate auditory hallucinations and delusions. It is an effective tool to track progress with schizophrenic clients and other clients with psychotic features. Examining 71 patients with diagnoses of schizophrenia or schizoaffective disorder, Haddock et al. (1999) reported median scores of 28 on the auditory hallucinations subscale (range = 14–39) and 15 on the delusions subscale (range = 5–22).

Rosenberg Self-Esteem Scale

This well-known instrument is both very brief and easy to administer, and has good psychometric properties. The scale measures global self-esteem (with higher total scores indicating greater self-esteem), so it is appropriate for use across a wide range of populations. We frequently use this tool as part of our assessment package for depressed clients.

To score, assign a value to each of the 10 items as follows, then total the scores: For items 1, 2, 4, 6, 7: Strongly Agree = 3, Agree = 2, Disagree = 1, and Strongly Disagree = 0. For items 3, 5, 8, 9, 10 (which are reversed in valence): Strongly Agree = 0, Agree = 1, Disagree = 2, and Strongly Disagree = 3. Thus, the possible range of responses is 0–30, with 30 indicating the highest self-esteem responses on all items.

This measure has been widely used, and different researchers often score the measure in different ways (e.g., 1–4 for each item rather than 0–3, or average rather than sum). Accordingly, the best way to find appropriate comparison norms for this scale is to search the literature for research using samples similar to your own.

The Rosenberg Self-Esteen Scale may be used without explicit permission. The author's family, however, would like to be kept informed of its use. Send information about how you have used the scale, or send published research resulting from its use, to the Morris Rosenberg Foundation, Department of Sociology, University of Maryland, 2112 Art/Soc Building, College Park, MD 20742-1315.

Yale–Brown Obsessive Compulsive Scale

The Y-BOCS is a helpful instrument for assessing progress in therapy for obsessive–compulsive disorder (OCD), because it indicates sensitivity to treatment and yields both a total severity score and separate obsession and compulsion subscale scores. The range of possible scores on each subscale is 0–20. Total Y-BOCS scores are calculated by summing the subscale scores. The 10-item clinician-administered scale measures the severity of obsessions and compulsions independent of the number and type of obsessions or compulsions present, making it a useful tool to monitor progress across clients with OCD, despite the heterogeneity of their symptoms.

As a comparison point, Table A.1 provides Y-BOCS subscale scores (Obsessions and Compulsions). The data in this table were taken from a treatment study involving 46 clients who received nine 90-minute weekly sessions of either live exposure and response prevention, or both live and imaginal exposure and response prevention (de Araujo, Ito, Marks, & Deale, 1995).

TABLE A.1. Means and Standard Deviations for the Y-BOCS across Brief Treatment

		Active treatment		Follow-up	
Subscale	Pretreatment	4 weeks	9 weeks	20 weeks	32 weeks
Obsessions					
ERP	14.7 (± 3.2)	9.4 (± 4.2)	7.6 (± 4.9)	9.0 (± 6.4)	8.6 (± 5.9)
ERP + imaginal	13.6 (± 2.7)	8.3 (± 2.5)	6.8 (± 3.6)	7.6 (± 4.4)	7.0 (± 3.0)
Compulsions					
ERP	14.1 (± 2.7)	10.5 (± 2.7)	7.9 (± 3.9)	8.8 (± 5.4)	8.0 (± 5.9)
ERP + imaginal	13.8 (± 2.1)	8.8 (± 2.3)	7.5 (± 3.2)	8.0 (± 4.0)	7.0 (± 2.9)

Note. ERP indicates live exposure and response prevention, and ERP + imaginal indicates both live and imaginal exposure and response prevention. These data were taken from de Araujo, Ito, Marks, and Deale (1995). Please see the original study for more details.

BRIEF PSYCHIATRIC RATING SCALE

Directions: Circle the appropriate number to represent level of severity of each symptom.

Scoring Criteria: 1 = Not Present 2 = Very Mild 3 = Mild 4 = Moderate
5 = Moderately Severe 6 = Severe 7 = Extremely Severe

1. SOMATIC CONCERN—preoccupation   1 2 3 4 5 6 7
   with physical health, fear of physical
   illness, hypochondriasis
2. ANXIETY—worry, fear, over-concern   1 2 3 4 5 6 7
   for present or future, uneasiness
3. EMOTIONAL WITHDRAWAL—lack of   1 2 3 4 5 6 7
   spontaneous interaction, isolation,
   deficiency in relating to others
4. CONCEPTUAL DISORGANIZATION—   1 2 3 4 5 6 7
   thought processes confused,
   disconnected, disorganized, disrupted
5. GUILT FEELINGS—self blame, shame,   1 2 3 4 5 6 7
   remorse for past behavior
6. TENSION—physical and motor   1 2 3 4 5 6 7
   manifestations of nervousness, over-
   activation
7. MANNERISMS AND POSTURING—   1 2 3 4 5 6 7
   peculiar, bizarre, unnatural motor
   behavior (not including tics)
8. GRANDIOSITY—exaggerated self-   1 2 3 4 5 6 7
   opinion, arrogance, conviction of
   unusual power or abilities
9. DEPRESSIVE MOOD—sorrow, sadness,   1 2 3 4 5 6 7
   despondency, pessimism
10. HOSTILITY—animosity, contempt,   1 2 3 4 5 6 7
    belligerence, disdain for others
11. SUSPICIOUSNESS—mistrust, belief   1 2 3 4 5 6 7
    others harbor malicious or
    discriminatory intent
12. HALLUCINATORY BEHAVIOR—   1 2 3 4 5 6 7
    perceptions without normal external
    stimulus correspondence

Reprinted with permission of authors and publisher from Overall, J. E., & Gorham, D. R. The brief psychiatric rating scale. *Psychological Reports*, 1962, *10*, 799–812. © Southern Universities Press, 1962.

13. MOTOR RETARDATION—slowed,   1 2 3 4 5 6 7
    weakened movements or speech,
    reduced body tone
14. UNCOOPERATIVENESS—resistance,   1 2 3 4 5 6 7
    guardedness, rejection of authority
15. UNUSUAL THOUGHT CONTENT—   1 2 3 4 5 6 7
    unusual, odd, strange, bizarre thought
    content
16. BLUNTED AFFECT—reduced   1 2 3 4 5 6 7
    emotional tone, reduction in formal
    intensity of feelings, flatness
17. EXCITEMENT—heightened emotional 1 2 3 4 5 6 7
    tone, agitation, increased reactivity
18. DISORIENTATION—confusion or lack 1 2 3 4 5 6 7
    of proper association for person, place,
    or time

BULIMIA TEST—REVISED

Directions: Answer each question by circling the number for the appropriate response. Please respond to each item as honestly as possible; remember all of the information you provide will be kept strictly confidential.

1. I am satisfied with my eating patterns.
   1. agree
   2. neutral
   3. disagree a little
   4. disagree
   5. disagree strongly

2. Would you presently call yourself a "binge eater"?
   1. yes, absolutely
   2. yes
   3. yes, probably
   4. yes, possibly
   5. no, probably not

3. Do you feel you have control over the amount of food you consume?
   1. most of the time
   2. a lot of the time
   3. occasionally
   4. rarely
   5. never

4. I am satisfied with the shape and size of my body.
   1. frequently or always
   2. sometimes
   3. occasionally
   4. rarely
   5. seldom or never

5. When I feel that my eating behavior is out of control, I try to take rather extreme measures to get back on course (strict dieting, fasting, laxatives, diuretics, self-induced vomiting, or vigorous exercise).
   1. always
   2. almost always
   3. frequently
   4. sometimes
   5. never or my eating behavior is never out of control

6. I use laxatives or suppositories to help control my weight.
    1. once a day or more
    2. 3–6 times a week
    3. once or twice a week
    4. 2–3 times a month
    5. once a month or less (or never)

7. I am obsessed about the size and shape of my body.
    1. always
    2. almost always
    3. frequently
    4. sometimes
    5. seldom or never

8. There are times when I rapidly eat a very large amount of food.
    1. more than twice a week
    2. twice a week
    3. once a week
    4. 2–3 times a month
    5. once a month or less (or never)

9. How long have you been binge eating (eating uncontrollably to the point of stuffing yourself)?
    1. not applicable; I don't binge eat
    2. less than 3 months
    3. 3 months–1 year
    4. 1–3 years
    5. 3 or more years

10. Most people I know would be amazed if they knew how much food I can consume at one sitting.
    1. without a doubt
    2. very probably
    3. probably
    4. possibly
    5. no

11. I exercise in order to burn calories.
    1. more than 2 hours per day
    2. about 2 hours per day
    3. more than 1 but less than 2 hours per day
    4. one hour or less per day
    5. I exercise but not to burn calories or I don't exercise

12. Compared with women your age, how preoccupied are you about your weight and body shape?
    1. a great deal more than average
    2. much more than average
    3. more than average
    4. a little more than average
    5. average or less than average

13. I am afraid to eat anything for fear that I won't be able to stop.
    1. always
    2. almost always
    3. frequently
    4. sometimes
    5. seldom or never

14. I feel tormented by the idea that I am fat or might gain weight.
    1. always
    2. almost always
    3. frequently
    4. sometimes
    5. seldom or never

15. How often do you intentionally vomit after eating?
    1. 2 or more times a week
    2. once a week
    3. 2–3 times a month
    4. once a month
    5. less than once a month or never

16. I eat a lot of food when I'm not even hungry.
    1. very frequently
    2. frequently
    3. occasionally
    4. sometimes
    5. seldom or never

17. My eating patterns are different from the eating patterns of most people.
    1. always
    2. almost always
    3. frequently
    4. sometimes
    5. seldom or never

18. After I binge eat I turn to one of several strict methods to try to keep from gaining weight (vigorous exercise, strict dieting, fasting, self-induced vomiting, laxatives, or diuretics).
    1. never or I don't binge eat
    2. rarely
    3. occasionally
    4. a lot of the time
    5. most or all of the time

19. I have tried to lose weight by fasting or going on strict diets.
    1. not in the past year
    2. once in the past year
    3. 2–3 times in the past year
    4. 4–5 times in the past year
    5. more than 5 times in the past year

20. I exercise vigorously and for long periods of time in order to burn calories.
    1. average or less than average
    2. a little more than average
    3. more than average
    4. much more than average
    5. a great deal more than average

21. When engaged in an eating binge, I tend to eat foods that are high in carbohydrates (sweets and starches).
    1. always
    2. almost always
    3. frequently
    4. sometimes
    5. seldom, or I don't binge

22. Compared to most people, my ability to control my eating behavior seems to be:
    1. greater than others' ability
    2. about the same
    3. less
    4. much less
    5. I have absolutely no control

23. I would presently label myself a "compulsive eater" (one who engages in episodes of uncontrolled eating).
    1. absolutely
    2. yes
    3. yes, probably
    4. yes, possibly
    5. no, probably not

24. I hate the way my body looks after I eat too much.
    1. seldom or never
    2. sometimes
    3. frequently
    4. almost always
    5. always

25. When I am trying to keep from gaining weight, I feel that I have to resort to vigorous exercise, strict dieting, fasting, self-induced vomiting, laxatives, or diuretics.
    1. never
    2. rarely
    3. occasionally
    4. a lot of the time
    5. most or all of the time

26. Do you believe that it is easier for you to vomit than it is for most people?
    1. yes, it's no problem at all for me
    2. yes, it's easier
    3. yes, it's a little easier
    4. about the same
    5. no, it's less easy

27. I use diuretics (water pills) to help control my weight.
    1. never
    2. seldom
    3. sometimes
    4. frequently
    5. very frequently

28. I feel that food controls my life.
    1. always
    2. almost always
    3. frequently
    4. sometimes
    5. seldom or never

29. I try to control my weight by eating little or no food for a day or longer.
    1. never
    2. seldom
    3. sometimes
    4. frequently
    5. very frequently

30. When consuming a large quantity of food, at what rate of speed do you usually eat?
    1. more rapidly than most people have ever eaten in their lives
    2. a lot more rapidly than most people
    3. a little more rapidly than most people
    4. about the same rate as most people
    5. more slowly than most people (or not applicable)

31. I use laxatives or suppositories to help control my weight.
    1. never
    2. seldom
    3. sometimes
    4. frequently
    5. very frequently

32. Right after I binge eat I feel:
    1. so fat and bloated I can't stand it
    2. extremely fat
    3. fat
    4. a little fat
    5. OK about how my body looks or I never binge eat

33. Compared to other people of my sex, my ability to always feel in control of how much I eat is:
    1. about the same or greater
    2. a little less
    3. less
    4. much less
    5. a great deal less

34. In the last 3 months, on the average how often did you binge eat (eat uncontrollably to the point of stuffing yourself)?
    1. once a month or less (or never)
    2. 2–3 times a month
    3. once a week
    4. twice a week
    5. more than twice a week

35. Most people I know would be surprised at how fat I look after I eat a lot of food.
    1. yes, definitely
    2. yes
    3. yes, probably
    4. yes, possibly
    5. no, probably not or I never eat a lot of food

36. I use diuretics (water pills) to help control my weight.
    1. 3 times a week or more
    2. once or twice a week
    3. 2–3 times a month
    4. once a month
    5. never

CENTER FOR EPIDEMIOLOGIC STUDIES— DEPRESSION SCALE (CES-D)

Directions: Below is a list of the ways you might have felt or behaved. Please circle the answer that best describes your situation *during the past week*:

0 = Rarely or none of the time (less than 1 day)
1 = Some or little of the time (1–2 days)
2 = Occasionally or a moderate amount of time (3–4 days)
3 = Most or all of the time (5–7 days)

DURING THE PAST WEEK:

1.	I was bothered by things that usually don't bother me.	0	1	2	3
2.	I did not feel like eating; my appetite was poor.	0	1	2	3
3.	I felt that I could not shake off the blues even with help from my family or friends.	0	1	2	3
4.	I felt that I was just as good as other people.	0	1	2	3
5.	I had trouble keeping my mind on what I was doing.	0	1	2	3
6.	I felt depressed.	0	1	2	3
7.	I felt that everything I did was an effort.	0	1	2	3
8.	I felt hopeful about the future.	0	1	2	3
9.	I thought my life had been a failure.	0	1	2	3
10.	I felt fearful.	0	1	2	3
11.	My sleep was restless.	0	1	2	3
12.	I was happy.	0	1	2	3
13.	I talked less than usual.	0	1	2	3
14.	I felt lonely.	0	1	2	3
15.	People were unfriendly.	0	1	2	3
16.	I enjoyed life.	0	1	2	3
17.	I had crying spells.	0	1	2	3
18.	I felt sad.	0	1	2	3
19.	I felt that people dislike me.	0	1	2	3
20.	I could not "get going."	0	1	2	3

From Radloff, L. S. (1977). The CES-D scale: A self-report depression scale for research in the general population. *Applied Psychological Measurement*, 1, 385–401. Reprinted with permission.

DAILY SPIRITUAL EXPERIENCES SCALE

Instructions: The list that follows includes items that you may or may not experience. Please consider how often you directly have this experience and try to disregard whether you feel you should or should not have these experiences. A number of items use the word "God." If this word is not a comfortable one, please substitute another word or thought that calls to mind the divine or holy for you.

	Many times a day	Every day	Most days	Some days	Once in awhile	Never or almost never
1. I feel God's presence.	1	2	3	4	5	6
2. I experience a connection to all of life.	1	2	3	4	5	6
3. I find strength in my religion or spirituality.	1	2	3	4	5	6
4. I feel God's love for me directly.	1	2	3	4	5	6
5. I feel God's love for me through others.	1	2	3	4	5	6
6. I ask for God's help in the midst of daily activities.	1	2	3	4	5	6
7. I feel guided by God in the midst of daily activities.	1	2	3	4	5	6
8. I feel deep inner peace or harmony.	1	2	3	4	5	6
9. I am fully present to life, not focused on the past or future.	1	2	3	4	5	6
10. During worship, or at other times when connecting with God, I feel intense joy which lifts me out of my daily concerns.	1	2	3	4	5	6
11. I am spiritually touched by the beauty of creation.	1	2	3	4	5	6
12. I feel thankful for my blessings.	1	2	3	4	5	6
13. I feel a selfless caring for others.	1	2	3	4	5	6
14. I accept others even when they do things I think are wrong.	1	2	3	4	5	6

Reprinted from Underwood, L. G. (1999). Daily Spiritual Experiences, *Multidimensional measurement of religiousness/spirituality for use in health research* (pp. 11–18), published by the John E. Fetzer Institute, Kalamazoo, MI. Public domain.

KANSAS MARITAL SATISFACTION SCALE

Directions: Please rate these three questions using the 1–7 scale below:
1 = Extremely Dissatisfied
2 = Very Dissatisfied
3 = Somewhat Dissatisfied
4 = Mixed
5 = Somewhat Satisfied
6 = Very Satisfied
7 = Extremely Satisfied

____ 1. How satisfied are you with your marriage?

____ 2. How satisfied are you with your husband [wife] as a spouse?

____ 3. How satisfied are you with your relationship with your husband [wife]?

Reprinted with permission from Schumm, W. R., Paff-Bergen, L. A., Hatch, R. C., Obiorah, F. C., Copeland, J. M., Meens, L. D., & Bugaighis, M. A. (1986). Concurrent and discriminant validity of the Kansas Marital Satisfaction Scale. *Journal of Marriage and the Family, 48*, 381–387.

PSYCHOTIC SYMPTOMS RATING SCALES

Auditory Hallucinations

A1 Frequency
0 Voices not present or present less than once a week
1 Voices occur at least once a week
2 Voices occur at least once a day
3 Voices occur at least once an hour
4 Voices occur continuously or almost continuously (i.e., stop for only a few minutes)

A2 Duration
0 Voices not present
1 Voices last for a few seconds, fleeting voices
2 Voices last for several minutes
3 Voices last for at least one hour
4 Voices last for hours

A3 Location
0 No voices present
1 Voices sound like they are inside head only
2 Voices outside the head, but close to ears/head; Voices inside head may also be present
3 Voices sound like they are inside or close to ears and outside head away from ears
4 Voices sound like they are from outside the head only

A4 Loudness
0 Voices not present
1 Quieter than own voice, whispers
2 About same loudness as own voice
3 Louder than own voice
4 Extremely loud, shouting

A5 Beliefs re: origin of voices
0 Voices not present
1 Believes voices to be solely internally generated and related to self
2 Holds 2% conviction that voices originate from external causes
3 Holds 50% conviction (but not 100%) that voices originate from external causes
4 Believes voices are solely due to external causes (100% conviction)

Reprinted with permission of Cambridge University Press and Dr. Gillian Haddock. This scale originally appeared in Haddock, G., McCarron, J., Tarrier, N., & Faragher, E. B. (1999). Scales to measure dimensions of hallucinations and delusions: The psychotic symptoms rating scales. *Psychological Medicine, 29,* 879–889.

A6 Amount of negative content of voices
0 No unpleasant content
1 Occasional unpleasant content (< 10%)
2 Minority of voice content is unpleasant or negative (< 50%)
3 Majority of voice content is unpleasant or negative (≥ 50%)
4 All of voice content is unpleasant or negative

A7 Degree of negative content
0 Not unpleasant or negative
1 Some degree of negative content, but not personal comments relating to self or family (e.g., swear words or comments not directed to self; e.g., "the milkman's ugly")
2 Personal verbal abuse, comments on behavior (e.g., "shouldn't do or say that")
3 Personal verbal abuse relating to self-concept (e.g., "you're lazy, ugly, mad, perverted")
4 Personal threats to self (e.g., threats to harm self or family, extreme instructions or commands to harm self or others)

A8 Amount of distress
0 Voices not distressing at all
1 Voices occasionally distressing, majority not distressing (< 10%)
2 Minority of voices distressing (< 50%)
3 Majority of voices distressing, minority not distressing (≥ 50%)
4 Voices always distressing

A9 Intensity of distress
0 Voices not distressing at all
1 Voices slightly distressing
2 Voices are distressing to a moderate degree
3 Voices are very distressing, although subject could feel worse
4 Voices are extremely distressing, feel the worst he/she could possibly feel

A10 Disruption to life caused by voices
0 No disruption to life, able to maintain social and family relationships (if present)
1 Voices cause minimal amount of disruption to life (e.g., interferes with concentration although able to maintain daytime activity and social and family relationships and able to maintain independent living without support)
2 Voices cause moderate amount of disruption to life causing some disturbance to daytime activity and/or family or social activities. The patient is not in hospital although may live in supported accommodation or receive additional help with daily living skills.

3 Voices cause severe disruption to life so that hospitalization is usually necessary. The patient is able to maintain some daily activities, self-care and relationships while in hospital. The patient may also be in supported accommodation but experiencing severe disruption of life in terms of activities, daily living skills, and/or relationships.

4 Voices cause complete disruption of daily life requiring hospitalization. The patient is unable to maintain any daily activities and social relationships. Self-care is also severely disrupted.

A11 Controllability of voices
0 Subject believes they can have control over the voices and can always bring on or dismiss them at will.
1 Subject believes they can have some control over the voices on the majority of occasions.
2 Subject believes they can have some control over their voices approximately half of the time.
3 Subject believes they can have some control over their voices but only occasionally. The majority of the time the subject experiences voices which are uncontrollable.
4 Subject has no control over when the voices occur and cannot dismiss or bring them on at all.

Delusions

B1 Amount of preoccupation with delusions
0 No delusions, or delusions which the subject thinks about less than once a week
1 Subject thinks about beliefs at least once a week
2 Subject thinks about beliefs at least once a day
3 Subject thinks about beliefs at least once an hour
4 Subject thinks about delusions continuously or almost continuously

B2 Duration of preoccupation with delusions
0 No delusions
1 Thoughts about beliefs last for a few seconds, fleeting thoughts
2 Thoughts about delusions last for several minutes
3 Thoughts about delusions last for at least 1 hour
4 Thoughts about delusions usually last for hours at a time

B3 Conviction
0 No conviction at all
1 Very little conviction in reality of beliefs, < 10%
2 Some doubts relating to conviction in beliefs, between 10–49%

3 Conviction in belief is very strong, between 50–99%
4 Conviction is 100%

B4 Amount of distress
0 Beliefs never cause distress
1 Beliefs cause distress on the minority of occasions
2 Beliefs cause distress on < 50% of occasions
3 Beliefs cause distress on the majority of occasions (50–99% of the time)
4 Beliefs always cause distress when they occur

B5 Intensity of distress
0 No distress
1 Beliefs cause slight distress
2 Beliefs cause moderate distress
3 Beliefs cause marked distress
4 Beliefs cause extreme distress, could not be worse

B6 Disruption to life caused by beliefs
0 No disruption to life, able to maintain independent living with no problems in daily living skills. Able to maintain social and family relationships (if present)
1 Beliefs cause minimal amount of disruption to life (e.g., interferes with concentration although able to maintain daytime activity and social and family relationships and be able to maintain independent living without support)
2 Beliefs cause moderate amount of disruption to life causing some disturbance to daytime activity and/or family or social activities. The patient is not in hospital although may live in supported accommodation or receive additional help with daily living skills.
3 Beliefs cause severe disruption to life so that hospitalization is usually necessary. The patient is able to maintain some daily activities, self-care and relationships while in hospital. The patient may also be in supported accommodation but experiencing severe disruption of life in terms of activities, daily living skills, and/or relationships.
4 Beliefs cause complete disruption of daily life requiring hospitalization. The patient is unable to maintain any daily activities and social relationships. Self-care is also severely disrupted.

ROSENBERG SELF-ESTEEM SCALE

Directions: Below is a list of statements dealing with your general feelings about yourself. If you strongly agree, circle SA. If you agree with the statement, circle A. If you disagree, circle D. If you strongly disagree, circle SD.

		Strongly Agree	Agree	Disagree	Strongly Disagree
1.	I feel that I am a person of worth, at least on an equal basis with others.	SA	A	D	SD
2.	I feel that I have a number of good qualities.	SA	A	D	SD
3.	All in all, I am inclined to feel that I am a failure.	SA	A	D	SD
4.	I am able to do things as well as most other people.	SA	A	D	SD
5.	I feel I do not have much to be proud of.	SA	A	D	SD
6.	I take a positive attitude toward myself.	SA	A	D	SD
7.	On the whole, I am satisfied with myself.	SA	A	D	SD
8.	I wish I could have more respect for myself.	SA	A	D	SD
9.	I certainly feel useless at times.	SA	A	D	SD
10.	At times I think I am no good at all.	SA	A	D	SD

YALE–BROWN OBSESSIVE COMPULSIVE SCALE (Y-BOCS)

Symptom Checklist

Check all that apply, but clearly mark the principal symptoms with a "P." (Rater must ascertain whether reported behaviors are bona fide symptoms of OCD, and not symptoms of another disorder such as simple phobia or hypochondriasis. Items marked as "*" may or may not be OCD phenomena.)

Current	Past	Aggressive obsessions
_____	_____	Fear might harm self
_____	_____	Fear might harm others
_____	_____	Violent or horrific images
_____	_____	Fear of blurting out obscenities or insults
_____	_____	Fear of doing something else embarrassing*
_____	_____	Fear will act on unwanted impulses (e.g., to stab friend)
_____	_____	Fear will steal things
_____	_____	Fear will harm others because not careful enough (e.g., hit/run car accident)
_____	_____	Fear will be responsible for something else terrible happening (e.g., fire, burglary)
_____	_____	Other _____

Current	Past	Contamination obsessions
_____	_____	Concerns or disgust with bodily waste or secretions (e.g., urine, feces, saliva)
_____	_____	Concerns with dirt or germs
_____	_____	Excessive concern with environmental contaminants (e.g., asbestos, radiation, toxic waste)
_____	_____	Excessive concern with household items (e.g., cleansers, solvents)
_____	_____	Excessive concern with animals (e.g., insects)
_____	_____	Bothered by sticky substances or residues
_____	_____	Concerned will get ill because of contaminant
_____	_____	Concerned will get others ill by spreading contaminant (aggressive)
_____	_____	No concern with consequences of contamination other than how it might feel
_____	_____	Other _____

Sexual obsessions

_____ _____ Forbidden or perverse sexual thoughts, images, or
impulses
_____ _____ Content involves children or incest
_____ _____ Content involves homosexuality*
_____ _____ Sexual behavior toward others (aggressive)*
_____ _____ Other _____

Hoarding/saving obsessions

[distinguish from hobbies and concern with objects
of monetary or sentimental value]

_____ _____ _____

Religious obsessions (scrupulosity)

_____ _____ Concerned with sacrilege and blasphemy
_____ _____ Excess concern with right/wrong, morality
_____ _____ Other _____

Obsession with need for symmetry or exactness

Accompanied by magical thinking (e.g., concerned
that mother will have accident unless things are in
_____ _____ the right place)
_____ _____ Not accompanied by magical thinking

Miscellaneous obsessions

_____ _____ Need to know or remember
_____ _____ Fear of saying certain things
_____ _____ Fear of not saying just the right thing*
_____ _____ Fear of losing things
_____ _____ Intrusive (nonviolent) images
_____ _____ Intrusive nonsense sounds, words, or music*
_____ _____ Bothered by certain sounds/noises*
_____ _____ Lucky/unlucky numbers
_____ _____ Colors with special significance
_____ _____ Superstitious fears
_____ _____ Other _____

Somatic obsessions

_____ _____ Concern with illness or disease*

Excessive concern with body part or aspect of
_____ _____ appearance (e.g., dysmorphophobia)*

_____ _____ Other _____

Cleaning/washing compulsions

_____ _____ Excessive or ritualized handwashing

Excessive or ritualized showering, bathing,
_____ _____ toothbrushing, grooming, or toilet routine

Involves cleaning of household items or other
_____ _____ inanimate objects

Other measures to prevent or remove contact with
_____ _____ contaminants

_____ _____ Other _____

Checking compulsions

_____ _____ Checking locks, stove, appliances, etc.

_____ _____ Checking that did not/will not harm others

_____ _____ Checking that did not/will not harm self

_____ _____ Checking that nothing terrible did/will happen

_____ _____ Checking that did not make mistake

_____ _____ Checking tied to somatic obsessions

_____ _____ Other _____

Repeating rituals

_____ _____ Rereading or rewriting

Need to repeat routine activities (e.g., in/out door,
_____ _____ up/down from chair)

_____ _____ Other _____

Counting compulsions

_____ _____ _____

Ordering/arranging compulsions

_____ _____ _____

<u>Hoarding/collecting compulsions</u>

[distinguish from hobbies and concern with objects of monetary or sentimental value (e.g., carefully reads junk mail, piles up old newspapers, sorts through garbage, collects useless objects)]

_____ _____ _____

<u>Miscellaneous compulsions</u>

_____	_____	Mental rituals (other than checking/counting)
_____	_____	Excessive listmaking
_____	_____	Need to tell, ask, or confess
_____	_____	Need to touch, tap, or rub*
_____	_____	Rituals involving blinking or staring*
_____	_____	Measures (not checking) to prevent harm to self, harm to others, or terrible consequences
_____	_____	Ritualized eating behaviors*
_____	_____	Superstitious behaviors
_____	_____	Trichotillomania*
_____	_____	Other self-damaging or self-mutilating behaviors*
_____	_____	Other _____

Yale–Brown Obsessive Compulsive Scale (Y-BOCS)

Y-BOCS TOTAL SCORE (add items 1–10) _____

	None	Mild	Moderate	Severe	Extreme
1. Time spent on obsessions	0	1	2	3	4

	No Symptoms	Long	Moderately Long	Short	Extremely Short
1b. Obsession-free interval (do not add to sub- total or total score)	0	1	2	3	4

	None	Mild	Moderate	Severe	Extreme
2. Interference from obsessions	0	1	2	3	4
3. Distress from obsessions	0	1	2	3	4

	Always Resists		Moderate		Completely Yields
4. Resistance	0	1	2	3	4

		Complete Control	Much Control	Moderate Control	Little Control	No Control
5.	Control over obsessions	0	1	2	3	4

Obsession subtotal (add items 1–5) ____

		None	Mild	Moderate	Severe	Extreme
6.	Time spent on compulsions	0	1	2	3	4

		No Symptoms	Long	Moderately Long	Short	Extremely Short
6b.	Compulsion-free interval (do not add to sub-total or total score)	0	1	2	3	4

		None	Mild	Moderate	Severe	Extreme
7.	Interference from compulsions	0	1	2	3	4
8.	Distress from compulsions	0	1	2	3	4

		Always Resists				Completely Yields
9.	Resistance	0	1	2	3	4

		Complete Control	Much Control	Moderate Control	Little Control	No Control
10.	Control over compulsions	0	1	2	3	4

Compulsion subtotal (add items 1–5) ____

		Excellent				Absent
11.	Insight into O–C symptoms	0	1	2	3	4

		None	Mild	Moderate	Severe	Extreme	
12.	Avoidance	0	1	2	3	4	
13.	Indecisiveness	0	1	2	3	4	
14.	Pathologic Responsibility	0	1	2	3	4	
15.	Slowness	0	1	2	3	4	
16.	Pathologic Doubting	0	1	2	3	4	
17.	Global Severity	0	1	2	3	4	5	6
18.	Global Improvement	0	1	2	3	4	5	6

19.	Reliability	Excellent = 0	Good = 1	Fair = 2	Poor = 3

SOURCES FOR OTHER MEASURES

Beck Depression Inventory and Beck Hopelessness Scale

Psychological Corporation (http://www.psychcorp.com) or (800) 872-1726
Both of these popular measures are available in several languages. The BDI is appropriate for adolescents and adults, and the BHS has been used for late adolescents and adults (17–80 years). They each take about 5 minutes to administer and 1 minute to score. Current pricing information is available on the website, but as of this writing, the prices were $33 for 25 copies or $126 for 100 copies. (All prices quoted in U.S. dollars.)

Behavior Assessment System for Children (BASC)

American Guidance Service (http://www.agsnet.com) or (800) 328-2560
This system for assessing children has the advantage of separate anxiety and depression scales (which some systems combine). Teacher and parent rating scales are available for evaluating children 2.5 to 18 years, and self-report scales are available for ages 8–18. The per-use price for hand-scored copies is a little more than $1.00 per copy, although the starter sets are more.

Brief Symptom Inventory (BSI)

The BSI is distributed by Clinical Psychometric Research, Inc. in Baltimore, Maryland. They can be reached by phone at (800) 245-0277 or by fax at (410) 321-6341. Their mailing address is P.O. Box 619, Riderwood, MD 21139.

Child Behavior Checklist (CBCL)

http://aseba.uvm.edu/index.html
Part of the Achenbach System of Empirically Based Assessment, the CBCL is a well-respected parent report of competencies and behavioral/emotional problems. There are separate versions for ages 4–18 and one for young adults 18–30 (and another for the wee ones 1.5–5 years).
The per-use cost is about $0.50 per copy for the hand-scored version, although the initial setup (buying the manuals, etc.) is an investment. Spanish versions are available.

Children's Depression Inventory (CDI)

Multi Health Systems (MHS; http://www.mhs.com) or (800) 456-3003 in the United States or (800) 268-6011 in Canada; fax: (888) 540-4484, e-mail: customerservice@mhs.com

This self-report scale has a first-grade reading level appropriate for children ages 7–17. Spanish and French versions are available, and the per-use cost is a little more than $1.00 per copy.

Conners' Rating Scales—Revised (CRS-R)

Multi Health Systems (MHS; http://www.mhs.com) or (800) 456-3003 in the United States or (800) 268-6011 in Canada; fax: (888) 540-4484, e-mail: *customerservice@mhs.com*

The Conners' scales are a widely used assessment of ADHD and oppositional behavior for children and adolescents ages 3–17. Spanish and French versions are available, and the system comes with versions for teacher-, parent-, and self-report. After the relatively costly initial setup, the per-use cost is a little more than $1.00 per copy.

Dyadic Adjustment Scale

Multi Health Systems (MHS) (http://www.mhs.com) or (800) 456-3003 in the United States or (800) 268-6011 in Canada, fax: (888) 540-4484, e-mail: *customerservice@mhs.com*

The DAS is a self-report measure (rated by an individual or a couple) of relationship adjustment along four dimensions: satisfaction, cohesion, consensus, and affection. The cost for 20 copies is $29.

RAND-36 Health Status Inventory

Psychological Corporation (http://www.psychcorp.com) or (800) 872-1726.

A 12-item version is also available. Representative, age-structured norms are available for ages 18–65. The price at the time of this writing is $8.00 for 25 copies.

Service Satisfaction Scale

This scale can be obtained from Dr. Greenfield at the Alcohol Research Group, 2000 Hearst Avenue, Berkeley, CA 94709; fax (510) 642-7175.

SHARP Consumer Satisfaction Scales

This scale was designed to measure consumer satisfaction with mental health services. The items cover services, the therapist, and treatment. The scale is scored for success, harmlessness, accessibility, respect, and partnership. A five-item validity scale is included to detect an unrealistically high level of satisfaction. This measure is archived in the Tests in Microfiche

Collection at the Educational Testing Service (ETS). Contact the ETS Test Collection Library at Rosedale and Carter Roads, Princeton, NJ 08541, or call them at (609) 734-5689. The document tracking number for this measure is TC014518.

Social Adjustment Scale—Self-Report

This measure is archived in the Tests in Microfiche Collection at the Educational Testing Service (ETS). Contact the ETS Test Collection Library at Rosedale and Carter Roads, Princeton, NJ 08541, or call them at (609) 734-5689. The document tracking number for this measure is TC007619.

Social Phobia and Anxiety Inventory (SPAI)

Multi Health Systems (MHS) (http://*www.mhs.com*) or (800) 456-3003 in the United States or (800) 268-6011 in Canada; fax: (888) 540-4484, e-mail: *customerservice@mhs.com*

The SPAI is a self-report measure assessing the somatic, cognitive, and behavioral symptoms of social phobia across a range of social situations. The cost for the manual plus 25 copies is $60. Subsequent administrations are $1.10 per copy.

REFERENCES

Adams, M., Palmer, A., Crook, W., & O'Brien, J. T. (2000). Health of the nation. Outcome scales for psychiatry: Are they valid? *Journal of Mental Health, 9*, 193–198.

Addis, M. E., Wade, W. A., & Hatgis, C. (1999). Barriers to dissemination of evidence-based practices: Addressing practitioners' concerns about manual-based psychotherapies. *Clinical Psychology: Science and Practice, 6*, 430–441.

American Psychiatric Association. (1993). Practice guideline for major depressive disorder in adults. *American Journal of Psychiatry, 150*(4, Suppl.), 1–26.

American Psychiatric Association. (1994). *Diagnostic and statistical manual of mental disorders* (4th ed.). Washington, DC: Author.

American Psychiatric Association. (1997). *Public mental health: A changing system in an era of managed care.* Washington, DC: Author.

Andrews, G., Peters, L., & Teesson, M. (1994). *Measurement of consumer outcomes. A report to the National Mental Health Information Strategy Committee of the Australian Health Ministers Advisory Council National Working Group on Mental Health Policy.*

Appel, C.-P. (1986). From contemplation to determination: Contributions from cognitive psychology. In W. R. Miller & N. Heather (Eds.), *Treating addictive behaviors: Processes of change. Applied clinical psychology* (pp. 59–89). New York: Plenum Press.

Bandura, A. (1977). Self-efficacy: Toward a unifying theory of behavioral change. *Psychological Review, 84*, 191–215.

Bandura, A., & Schunk, D. H. (1981). Cultivating competence, self-efficacy, and intrinsic interest through proximal self-motivation. *Journal of Personality and Social Psychology, 41,* 586–598.

Bandura, A., & Simon, K. M. (1977). The role of proximal intentions in self-regulation of refractory behavior. *Cognitive Therapy and Research, 1,* 177–193.

Bartlett, J. (1997). Treatment outcomes: The psychiatrist's and health care executive's perspectives. *Psychiatric Annals, 27*(2), 100–103.

Beck, A. T., Weissman, A., Lester, D., & Trexler, L. (1974). The measurement of pessimism: The Hopelessness Scale. *Journal of Consulting and Clinical Psychology, 42*(6), 861–865.

Beitman, B. D., Goldfried, M. R., & Norcross, J. C. (1989). The movement toward integrating the psychotherapies: An overview. *American Journal of Psychiatry, 146,* 138–147.

Bergin, A. E., & Garfield, S. L. (Eds.). (1994). *Handbook of psychotherapy and behavior change* (4th ed.). New York: Wiley.

Bernstein, S. (1992). A protocol illustrating a competency-based approach to cognitive therapy. *Psychotherapy, 29,* 269–273.

Beutler, L. E., & Harwood, T. M. (1995). Prescriptive psychotherapies. *Applied and Preventive Psychology, 4,* 89–100.

Brehm, S. S., & Smith, T. W. (1986). Social psychological approaches to psychotherapy and behavior change. In S. L. Garfield & A. E. Bergin (Eds.), *Handbook of psychotherapy and behavior change* (3rd ed., pp. 69–115). New York: Wiley.

Brickman, P., Rabinowitz, V. C., Karuza, J., Coates, D., Cohn, E., & Kidder, L. (1982). Models of helping and coping. *American Psychologist, 37*(4), 368–384.

Bruch, M., & Bond, F. W. (Eds.). (1998). *Beyond diagnosis: Case formulation approaches in CBT.* Chichester, UK: Wiley.

Budman, S. H., & Gurman, A. S. (1988). *Theory and practice of brief psychotherapy.* New York: Guilford Press.

Carr, J. E., & Burkholder, E. O. (1998). Creating single subject design graphs with Microsoft Excel™. *Journal of Applied Behavior Analysis, 31,* 245–251.

Cavior, N., & Marabotto, C. M. (1976). Monitoring verbal behaviors in a dyadic interaction. *Journal of Consulting and Clinical Psychology, 44*(1), 68–76.

Chamberlain, P., Patterson, G., Reid, J., Kavanagh, K., & Forgatch, M. (1984). Observation of client resistance. *Behavior Therapy, 15,* 144–155.

Chambless, D. L., Baker, M. J., Baucom, D. H., Beutler, L. E., Calhoun, K. S., Crits-Christoph, P., Daiuto, A., DeRubeis, R., Detweiler, J., Haaga, D. A. F., Bennett Johnson, S., McCurry, S., Mueser, K. T., Pope, K. S., Sanderson, W. C., Shoham, V., Stickle, T., Williams, D. A., & Woody, S. R.

(1998). Update on empirically validated therapies, II. *The Clinical Psychologist, 51*(1), 3–16.

Chambless, D. L., Caputo, G. C., Jasin, S. E., Gracely, E. J., & Williams, C. (1985). The Mobility Inventory for agoraphobia. *Behaviour Research and Therapy, 23*, 33–44.

Chen, H. (1993). Emerging perspectives in program evaluation. *Journal of Social Service Research, 17*(1/2), 1–17.

Cho, M., Moscicki, E., Narrow, W., Rae, D., Locke, B., & Regier, A. (1993). Concordance between two measures of depression in the Hispanic Health and Nutrition Examination Survey. *Social Psychiatry and Psychiatric Epidemiology, 28*, 156–163.

Craske, M. G., Meadows, E. A., & Barlow, D. H. (1994). *Mastery of your anxiety and Panic II and agoraphobia supplement: Therapist Guide.* San Antonio: Psychological Corporation.

Dana, R. H. (1993). *Multicultural assessment perspectives for professional psychologists.* Needham Heights, MA: Allyn & Bacon.

Dawes, R. M. (1994). *House of cards: Psychology and psychotherapy built on myth.* New York: Free Press.

de Araujo, L. A., Ito, L. M., Marks, I. M., & Deale, E. (1995). Does imagined exposure to the consequence of not ritualising enhance live exposure for OCD? A controlled study: I. Main outcome. *British Journal of Psychiatry, 167*, 65–70.

Derogatis, L. R., & Melisaratos, N. (1983). The Brief Symptom Inventory: An introductory report. *Psychological Medicine, 13*(3), 595–605.

DiClemente, C. C. (1991). Motivational interviewing and the stages of change. In W. R. Miller & S. Rollnick (Eds.), *Motivational interviewing: Preparing people to change addictive behavior* (pp. 191–202). New York: Guilford Press.

DiClemente, C. C., Prochaska, J. O., Fairhurst, S. K., Velicer, W. F., Velasquez, M. M., & Rossi, J. S. (1991). The process of smoking cessation: An analysis of precontemplation, contemplation, and preparation stages of change. *Journal of Consulting and Clinical Psychology, 59*, 295–304.

DiClemente, C. C., Prochaska, J. O., & Gilbertini, M. (1985). Self-efficacy and the stages of self-change of smoking. *Cognitive Therapy and Research, 9*, 181–200.

Dingemans, P. M., Winter, M. L. F., Bleeker, J. A. C., & Rathod, P. (1983). A cross-cultural study of the reliability and factorial dimensions of the Brief Psychiatric Rating Scale (BPRS). *Psychopharmacology, 80*, 190–191.

D'Zurilla, T. J. (1986). *Problem-solving therapy: A social competence approach to clinical intervention.* New York: Springer.

Eells, T. (1997). Psychotherapy case formulation: History and current status. In T. Eells (Ed.), *Handbook of psychotherapy case formulation* (pp. 1–25). New York: Guilford Press.

Eisen, S. V., Dill, D. L., & Grob, M. C. (1994). Reliability and validity of a brief patient-report instrument for psychiatric outcome evaluation. *Hospital and Community Psychiatry, 45,* 242–247.

Eisenberg, G. M. (1981). Midtherapy training: Extending the present system of pretherapy training. *Dissertation Abstracts International, 41,* 2754B.

English, H. B., & English, A. C. (1958). *A comprehensive dictionary of psychological and psychoanalytic terms.* New York: McKay.

Eysenck, H. J. (1970). A mish-mash of theories. *International Journal of Psychiatry, 9,* 140–146.

Falk, L. (1999). Development and first results of the Borderline Personality Inventory: A self-report instrument for assessing borderline personality organization. *Journal of Personality Assessment, 73,* 45–63.

Fiske, S., & Taylor, S. E. (1984). *Social cognition.* Reading, MA: Addison-Wesley.

Forquer, S. L., & Muse, L. C. (1996). Continuous quality improvement: Theory and tools for the 1990s. In B. L. Levin & J. Petrila (Eds.), *Mental health services: A public health perspective.* New York: Oxford University Press.

Friedlander, M. L. (1981). The effects of delayed role induction on counseling process and outcome. *Dissertation Abstracts International, 43,* 3887B–3888B.

Gabbard, G. O. (Ed.). (2001). *Treatments of psychiatric disorders* (3rd ed.). Washington, DC: American Psychiatric Press.

Galasso, D. (1987). Guidelines for developing multidisciplinary treatment plans. *Hospital and Community Psychiatry, 38,* 394–397.

Gambrill, E. (1999). Evidence-based practice: An alternative to authority-based practice. *Families in Society: The Journal of Contemporary Human Services, 80,* 341–350.

Garb, H. N. (1994). Cognitive heuristics and biases in personality assessment. In L. Heath, R. S. Tindale, J. Edwards, E. J. Posavac, F. B. Bryant, E. Henderson-King, Y. Suarez-Balcazar, & J. Myers (Eds.), *Applications of heuristics and biases to social issues* (pp. 73–90). New York: Plenum Press.

Garfield, S. L. (1996). Some problems associated with "validated" forms of psychotherapy. *Clinical Psychology Science and Practice, 3,* 218–229.

Glazer, W. M. (1994). What are "best practices"?: Understanding the concept. *Hospital and Community Psychiatry, 45,* 1067–1068.

Goldberg, L. R. (1959). The effectiveness of clinicians' judgments: The diagnosis of organic brain damage from the Bender Gestalt Test. *Journal of Consulting Psychology, 23,* 25–33.

Goldfried, M. R. (1980). Toward the delineation of therapeutic change principles. *American Psychologist, 35,* 991–999.

Goldfried, M. R., & Davison, G. C. (1994). *Clinical behavior therapy* (expanded ed.). New York: Wiley.

Golding, J. M., & Burnam, M. A. (1990). Immigration, stress, and depressive symptoms in a Mexican-American community. *Journal of Nervous and Mental Disease, 178,* 161–171.

Goldstein, A., & Stein, N. (1976). *Prescriptive psychotherapies.* New York: Pergamon Press.

Goodman, W. K., Price, L. H., Rasmussen, S. A., Mazure, C., Fleischmann, R. L., Hill, C. L., Heninger, G. R., & Charney, D. S. (1989). Yale–Brown Obsessive Compulsive Scale: I. Development, use, and reliability. *Archives of General Psychiatry, 46,* 1006–1011.

Gottman, J. M., & Leiblum, S. R. (1974). *How to do psychotherapy and how to evaluate it: A manual for beginners.* New York: Holt, Rinehart & Winston.

Greenfield, T. K., & Attkisson, C. C. (1989). Steps toward a multifactorial satisfaction scale for primary care and mental health services. *Evaluation and Program Planning, 12,* 271–278.

Gunderson, J. G. (1984). *Borderline personality disorder.* Washington, DC: American Psychiatric Press.

Haaga, D. A. F. (2000). Introduction to the special section on stepped care models in psychotherapy. *Journal of Consulting and Clinical Psychology, 68,* 547–548.

Haas, L. J., & Cummings, N. A. (1991). Managed outpatient mental health plans: Clinical, ethical, and practical guidelines for participation. *Professional Psychology, 22,* 45–51.

Haddock, G., McCarron, J., Tarrier, N., & Faragher, E. B. (1999). Scales to measure dimensions of hallucinations and delusions: The psychotic symptoms rating scales. *Psychological Medicine, 29,* 879–889.

Hammond, W. R., & Yung, B. (1993). Minority student recruitment and retention practices among schools of professional psychology: A national survey and analysis. *Professional Psychology: Research and Practice, 24,* 3–12.

Hartshorne, H., & May, M. A. (1928). *Studies in the nature of character: Vol. 1. Studies in deceit.* New York: Macmillan.

Havik, O. E., & VandenBos, G. R. (1996). Limitations of manualized psychotherapy for everyday clinical practice. *Clinical Psychology Science and Practice, 3,* 264–267.

Hayes, S. C., Barlow, D. H., & Nelson-Gray, R. O. (1999). *The scientist practitioner: Research and accountability in the age of managed care* (2nd ed.). Boston, MA: Allyn & Bacon.

Hays, P. A. (1995). Multicultural applications of cognitive-behavior therapy. *Professional Psychology: Research and Practice, 26*(3), 309–315.

Heinssen, R. K., Levendusky, P. G., & Hunter, R. H. (1995). Client as colleague: Therapeutic contracting with the seriously mentally ill. *American Psychologist, 50*, 522–532.

Henry, W. P. (1997). Conceptual issues in measuring personality disorder change. In H. H. Strupp & L. M. Horowitz (Eds.), *Measuring patient changes in mood, anxiety, and personality disorders: Toward a core battery* (pp. 461–488). Washington, DC: American Psychological Association.

Hollenbeck, J. R., Williams, C. R., & Klein, H. J. (1989). An empirical examination of the antecedents of commitment to difficult goals. *Journal of Applied Psychology, 74*, 18–23.

Janis, I. L., & Mann, L. (1977). *Decision making: A psychological analysis of conflict, choice, and commitment.* New York: Free Press.

Kazdin, A. E. (1998). *Research design in clinical psychology* (3rd ed.). Boston: Allyn & Bacon.

Keisler, C. A. (2000). The next wave of change for psychology and mental health services in the health care revolution. *American Psychologist, 55*, 481–487.

Kirk, S. A. (1999). Good intentions are not enough: Practice guidelines for social work. *Research on Social Work Practice, 9*, 302–310.

Koenigsberg, H. W., Kaplan, R. D., Gilmore, M. M., & Cooper, A. M. (1985). The relationship between syndrome and personality disorder in DSM-III: Experience with 2,462 patients. *American Journal of Psychiatry, 142*, 207–212.

Lambert, M. J. (1994). Use of psychological tests for outcome assessment. In M. E. Maruish (Ed.), *The use of psychological testing for treatment planning and outcome assessment.* (pp. 75–97). Hillsdale, NJ: Erlbaum.

Lambert, M. J., Okiishi, J. C., Finch, A. E., & Johnson, L. D. (1998). Outcome assessment: From conceptualization to implementation. *Professional Psychology: Research and Practice, 29*, 63–70.

Lazarus, A. A. (1997). *Brief but comprehensive psychotherapy: The multimodal way.* New York: Springer.

Lazarus, A. A., Beutler, L. E., & Norcross, J. C. (1992). The future of technical eclecticism. *Psychotherapy, 29*, 11–20.

Lewis, J. M., & Usdin, G. (1982). *Treatment planning in psychiatry.* Washington, DC: American Psychiatric Association.

Lichtenstein, E. (1982). The smoking problem: A behavioral perspective. *Journal of Consulting and Clinical Psychology, 50*(6), 804–819.

Linehan, M. M. (1993). *Cognitive-behavioral treatment of borderline personality disorder.* New York: Guilford Press.

Livingston, R. (1999). Cultural issues in diagnosis and treatment of ADHD.

Journal of the American Academy of Child and Adolescent Psychiatry, 38, 1591–1594.

Locke, E. A., Shaw, K. N., Saari, L. M., & Latham, G. P. (1981). Goal setting and task performance: 1969–1980. *Psychological Bulletin, 90,* 125–152.

Lopez, S. R. (1989). Patient variable biases in clinical judgment: Conceptual overview and methodological considerations. *Psychological Bulletin, 106*(2), 184–203.

Lopez, S. R. (1997). Cultural competence in psychotherapy: A guide for clinicians and their supervisors. In C. E. Watkins, Jr. (Ed.), *Handbook of psychotherapy supervision* (pp. 570–588). New York: Wiley.

Loranger, A. W. (1990). The impact of DSM-III on diagnostic practice in a university hospital: A comparison of DSM-II and DSM-III in 10,914 patients. *Archives of General Psychiatry, 47,* 672–675.

Luborsky, L., Crits-Cristoph, P., Mintz, J., & Auerbach, A. (1988). *Who will benefit from psychotherapy? Predicting therapeutic outcomes.* New York: Basic Books.

Luborsky, L., McLellan, A. T., Woody, G. E., O'Brien, C. P., & Auerbach, A. (1985). Therapist success and its determinants. *Archives of General Psychiatry, 42,* 602–611.

Luepnitz, R. R., Randolph, D. L., & Gutsch, K. U. (1982). Race and socioeconomic status as confounding variables in the accurate diagnosis of alcoholism. *Journal of Clinical Psychology, 38*(3), 665–669.

Lyons, J. S., Howard, K. I., O'Mahoney, M. T., & Lish, J. D. (1997). *The measurement and management of clinical outcomes in mental health.* New York: Wiley.

Makover, R. B. (1992). Training psychotherapists in hierarchical treatment planning. *Journal of Psychotherapy Practice and Research, 1,* 337–350.

Makover, R. B. (1996). *Treatment planning for psychotherapists.* Washington, DC: American Psychiatric Press.

Marlatt, G. A., & Gordon, J. R. (Eds.). (1985). *Relapse prevention: Maintenance strategies in the treatment of addictive behaviors.* New York: Guilford Press.

Masterson, J. (1972). *Treatment of the borderline adolescent: A developmental approach.* New York: Wiley.

Mattaini, M. A. (1993). *More than a thousand words: Graphics for clinical practice.* Washington, DC: NASW Press.

McConnaughy, E. A., DiClemente, C. C., Prochaska, J. O., & Velicer, W. F. (1989). Stages of change in psychotherapy: A follow-up report. *Psychotherapy, 26,* 494–503.

McCrady, B. S. (1993). Alcoholism. In D. H. Barlow (Ed.), *Clinical handbook of psychological disorders* (2nd ed.). New York: Guilford Press.

McHorney, C. A., Ware, J. E., & Raczek, A. E. (1993). The MOS 36–item

Short-Form Health Survey (SF-36): II. Psychometric and clinical tests of validity in measuring physical and mental health constructs. *Medical Care, 31,* 247–263.

Meehl, P. E. (1973). Why I do not attend case conferences. In P. E. Meehl (Ed.), *Psychodiagnosis: Selected papers* (pp. 225–302). Minneapolis: University of Minnesota Press.

Miller, W. R. (1985). Motivation for treatment: A review with special emphasis on alcoholism. *Psychological Bulletin, 98*(1), 84–107.

Miller, W. R. (Ed.). (1999). *Integrating spirituality into treatment: Resources for practitioners.* Washington, DC: American Psychological Association.

Miller, W. R., & Rollnick, S. (1991). *Motivational interviewing: Preparing people to change addictive behavior.* New York: Guilford Press.

Miller, W. R., & Sovereign, R. G. (1989). The check-up: A model for early intervention in addictive behaviors. In T. Loberg & W. R. Miller (Eds.), *Addictive behaviors: Prevention and early intervention* (pp. 219–231). Amsterdam, Netherlands: Swets & Zeitlinger.

Mischel, W. (1968). *Personality and assessment.* New York: Wiley.

Morgan, D. L., & Morgan, R. K. (2001). Single-participant research design: Bringing science to managed care. *American Psychologist, 56,* 119–127.

Morrison, J. K. (1984). Crossing the research barrier in the private practice of psychotherapy. *Psychotherapy in Private Practice, 2*(3), 15–20.

Nathan, P. E., & Gorman, J. M. (Eds.). (2002). *A guide to treatments that work* (2nd ed.). New York: Oxford University Press.

Nelson, R. O. (1981). Realistic dependent measures for clinical use. *Journal of Consulting and Clinical Psychology, 49,* 168–182.

Newman, C. F. (1994). Understanding client resistance: Methods for enhancing motivation to change. *Cognitive and Behavioral Practice, 1*(1), 47–69.

Newman, C. F. (1996). A cognitive perspective on resistance in psychotherapy. *In Session: Psychotherapy in Practice, 2*(1), 33–43.

Norcross, J. C., & Vangarelli, D. J. (1989). The resolution solution: Longitudinal examination of New Year's change attempts. *Journal of Substance Abuse, 1*(2), 127–134.

Nossiter, J. C. (1995). *Using Excel 5 for Windows.* Indianapolis, IN: Que Corporation.

Ogles, B. M., Lambert, M. J., & Masters, K. S. (1996). *Assessing outcome in clinical practice.* Boston: Allyn & Bacon.

O'Keefe, J., Quittner, A. L., & Melamed, B. (1996). Quality and outcome indicators. In R. L. Glueckauf, R. G. Frank, G. R. Bond & J. H. McGrew (Eds.), *Psychological practice in a changing health care system: Issues and new directions* (pp. 134–149). New York: Springer.

O'Leary, K. D., & Wilson, G. T. (1987). *Behavior therapy: Application and outcome.* Englewood Cliffs, NJ: Prentice-Hall.

Organista, K. C., & Muñoz, R. F. (1996). Cognitive-behavioral therapy with Latinos. *Cognitive and Behavioral Practice, 3,* 255–270.

Overall, J. E., & Gorham, D. R. (1962). The Brief Psychiatric Rating Scale. *Psychological Reports, 10,* 799–812.

Patterson, C. H. (1989). Foundations for a systematic eclectic psychotherapy. *Psychotherapy, 26,* 427–435.

Paul, G. L. (1974). Experimental–behavioral approaches to "schizophrenia." In R. Cancro, N. Fox, & L. E. Shapiro (Eds.), *Strategic intervention in schizophrenia: Current developments in treatment* (pp. 187–200). New York: Behavioral Publications.

Persons, J., & Tompkins, M. (1997). Cognitive-behavioral case formulation. In T. Eells (Ed.), *Handbook of psychotherapy case formulation* (pp. 314–339). New York: Guilford Press.

Persons, J. B. (1989). *Cognitive therapy in practice: A case formulation approach.* New York: Norton.

Peterson, R. A., & Reiss, S. (1987). *Anxiety Sensitivity Index manual.* Palos Heights, IL: International Diagnostic Systems.

Prochaska, J. O. (1991). Prescribing to the stages and levels of change. *Psychotherapy, 28,* 463–468.

Prochaska, J. O., & DiClemente, C. C. (1982). Transtheoretical therapy: Toward a more integrative model of change. *Psychotherapy: Theory, Research and Practice, 19*(3), 276–288.

Prochaska, J. O., & DiClemente, C. C. (1984). *The transtheoretical approach: Crossing traditional boundaries of change.* Homewood, IL: Dorsey Press.

Prochaska, J. O., & DiClemente, C. C. (1992). The transtheoretical approach. In J. C. Norcross & M. R. Goldfried (Eds.), *Handbook of psychotherapy integration* (pp. 300–334). New York: Basic Books.

Prochaska, J. O., DiClemente, C. C., & Norcross, J. C. (1992). In search of how people change: Applications to addictive behaviors. *American Psychologist, 47*(9), 1102–1114.

Putnam, D. E., Finney, J. W., Barkley, P. L., & Bonner, M. J. (1994). Enhancing commitment improves adherence to a medical regimen. *Journal of Consulting and Clinical Psychology, 62,* 191–194.

Quality Assurance Project. (1982). A treatment outline for agoraphobia. *Australian and New Zealand Journal of Psychiatry, 16,* 25–33.

Quality Assurance Project. (1985). Treatment outlines for the management of obsessive–compulsive disorders. *Australian and New Zealand Journal of Psychiatry, 19,* 240–253.

Radloff, L. S. (1977). The CES-D scale: A self-report depression scale for research in the general population. *Applied Psychological Measurement, 1,* 385–401.

Rhoades, H. M., & Overall, J. E. (1988). The semi-structured BPRS interview and rating guide. *Psychopharmacology Bulletin, 24,* 101–104.

Roberts, R. (1980). Reliability of the CES-D scale in different ethnic contexts. *Psychiatry Research, 2,* 125–134.

Rogers, C. R. (1958). A process conception of psychotherapy. *American Psychologist, 13,* 142–149.

Rogler, L. H., Malgady, R. G., Costantino, G., & Blumenthal, R. (1987). What do culturally sensitive mental health services mean?: The case of Hispanics. *American Psychologist, 42,* 565–570.

Rosen, L. D., & Weil, M. M. (1996). Easing the transition from paper to computer-based systems. In T. Trabin (Ed.), *The computerization of behavioral healthcare: How to enhance clinical practice, management, and communications* (pp. 87–107). San Francisco: Jossey-Bass.

Rosenberg, M. (1962). The association between self-esteem and anxiety. *Journal of Psychiatric Research, 1,* 135–152.

Ryder, A. G., Alden, L. E., & Paulhus, D. L. (2000). Is acculturation unidimensional or bidimensional?: A head-to-head comparison in the prediction of personality, self-identity, and adjustment. *Journal of Personality and Social Psychology, 79,* 49–65.

Sackett, D. L., Richardson, W. S., Rosenberg, W., & Haynes, R. B. (1997). *Evidence-based medicine: How to practice and teach EBM.* Oxford, UK: Oxford University Press.

Schumm, W. R., Paff-Bergen, L. A., Hatch, R. C., Obiorah, F. C., Copeland, J. M., Meens, L. D., & Bugaighis, M. A. (1986). Concurrent and discriminant validity of the Kansas Marital Satisfaction Scale. *Journal of Marriage and the Family, 48,* 381–387.

Sederer, L. I., & Dickey, B. (Eds.). (1996). *Outcomes assessment in clinical practice.* Baltimore, MD: Williams & Wilkins.

Shaffer, I. A. (1997). Treatment outcomes: Economic and ethical considerations. *Psychiatric Annals, 27*(2), 104–107.

Sieck, W. A., & McFall, R. M. (1976). Some determinants of self-monitoring effects. *Journal of Consulting and Clinical Psychology, 44*(6), 958–965.

Sperry, L., Gudeman, J. E., Blackwell, B., & Faulkner, L. R. (1992). *Psychiatric case formulations.* Washington, DC: American Psychiatric Association.

Stephenson, M. (2000). Development and validation of the Stephenson Multigroup Acculturation Scale (SMAS). *Psychological Assessment, 12,* 77–88.

Strupp, H. H., Horowitz, L. M., & Lambert, M. J. (Eds.). (1997). *Measuring patient changes in mood, anxiety, and personality disorders: Toward a core battery.* Washington, DC: American Psychological Association.

Sue, S. (1998). In search of cultural competence in psychotherapy and counseling. *American Psychologist, 53,* 440–448.

Sue, S., & Zane, N. (1987). The role of culture and cultural techniques in psychotherapy: A critique and reformulation. *American Psychologist,* 42, 37–45.

Tanner, B. A. (1982). A multi-dimensional client satisfaction instrument. *Evaluation and Program Planning, 5,* 161–167.

Tanner, B. A., & Stacey, W. (1985). A validity scale for the SHARP Consumer Satisfaction Scales. *Evaluation and Program Planning, 8,* 147–153.

Thelen, M. H., Farmer, J., Wonderlich, S., & Simi, M. (1991). A revision of the Bulimia Test: The BULIT-R. *Psychological Assessment: A Journal of Consulting and Clinical Psychology, 3,* 119–124.

Turkat, I. (1985). *Behavioral case formulation.* Cambridge, MA: Perseus.

Turner, R., & Dudek, P. (1997). Outcome evaluation of psychosocial treatment for personality disorders: Functions, obstacles, goals, and strategies. In H. H. Strupp, L. M. Horowitz, & M. J. Lambert (Eds.), *Measuring patient changes in mood, anxiety, and personality disorders: Toward a core battery* (pp. 433–460). Washington, DC: American Psychological Association.

Underwood, L. G. (1999). *Daily spiritual experiences: Multidimensional measurement of religiousness/spirituality for use in health research* (pp. 11–18). Kalamazoo, MI: John E. Fetzer Institute.

Vallis, T. M., Shaw, B. F., & Dobson, K. S. (1986). The Cognitive Therapy Scale: Psychometric properties. *Journal of Consulting and Clinical Psychology, 54*(3), 381–385.

Volkman, V. D. (1987). *Six steps in the treatment of borderline personality organization.* Northvale, NJ: Jason Aronson.

Ware, J. E., & Sherbourne, C. D. (1992). The MOS 36–item Short-Form Health Survey (SF-36): I. Conceptual framework and item selection. *Medical Care, 30,* 473–483.

Webster's New Collegiate Dictionary (9th ed.). (1983). Springfield, MA: Merriam-Webster.

Weissman, M. M., & Bothwell, S. (1976). The assessment of social adjustment by patients self-report. *Archives of General Psychiatry, 33,* 1111–1115.

Whiston, S. C., & Sexton, T. L. (1993). An overview of psychotherapy outcome research: Implications for practice. *Professional Psychology: Research and Practice, 24,* 43–51.

Wiggins, J. S. (1973). *Personality and prediction: Predictors of personality assessment.* Reading, MA: Addison-Wesley.

Wilson, G. T. (1985). Psychological prognostic factors in the treatment of obesity. In J. Hirsch & T. B. Van Itallie (Eds.), *Recent advances in obesity research* (Vol. 4, pp. 301–311). London: Libbey.

Wilson, G. T. (1998). Manual-based treatment and clinical practice. *Clinical Psychology: Science and Practice, 5,* 363–375.

Wilson, P. H. (Ed.). (1992). *Principles and practice of relapse prevention*. New York: Guilford Press.

Zanarini, M. C., & Frankenburg, F. R. (1994). Emotional hypochondriasis, hyperbole, and the borderline patient. *Journal of Psychotherapy Practice and Research, 3,* 25–36.

Zimmerman, M. (1994). Diagnosing personality disorders: A review of issues and research methods. *Archives of General Psychiatry, 51,* 225–245.

INDEX

Accountability
  definition, 6
  enhancement of, 6, 7
Acculturation, 30, 31
Alcohol use/abuse
  assessment, 35, 36, 92, 95
  relapse prevention, 163, 164
Anger management
  decision tree, case study, 175-188
  diary record, 89, 177-180
Anxiety disorders
  measurement, 108, 109
  multimodal assessment, case
      study, 110-113
Assertiveness skills, checklist, 107,
      108
Assertiveness training
  case study, 176-178
  cultural considerations, 152
Assessment (*see* Measurement)
"Autofill," 132, 133
Axis II conditions (*see* Personality
      disorders)

B

Baseline data
  case examples, 139, 140, 180, 181
  collection challenges, 127, 128
  graphing, 125-128, 133, 134, 139, 140
  principle features, 125, 126
BASIC-ID model, 34
BASIS-32, 100, 101
Beck Depression Inventory, 230
Behavior and Symptom
      Identification Scale, 100, 102
Behavior Assessment System for
      Children, 99, 230
Behavioral assessment, social
      phobia, 111-113
Behavioral change
  decisional balance, 161, 262
  graphing, 136, 137
  maintenance of, 164, 165
  motivation for, 78-80, 161-163
  ongoing measurement, 98, 99
  stage model, 79